Recent Advances in Cesarean Delivery

Edited by Georg Schmölzer

Published in London, United Kingdom

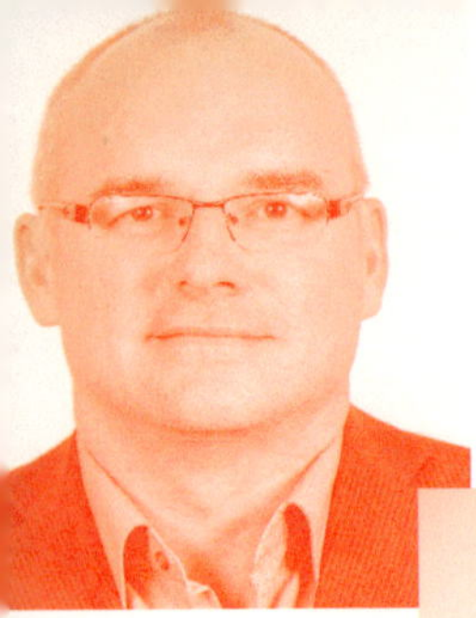
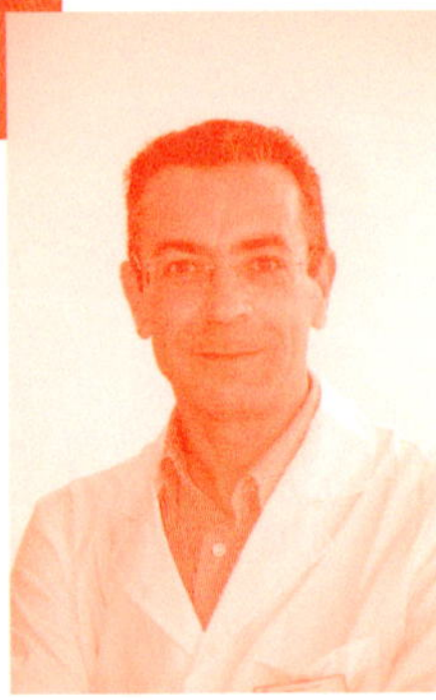
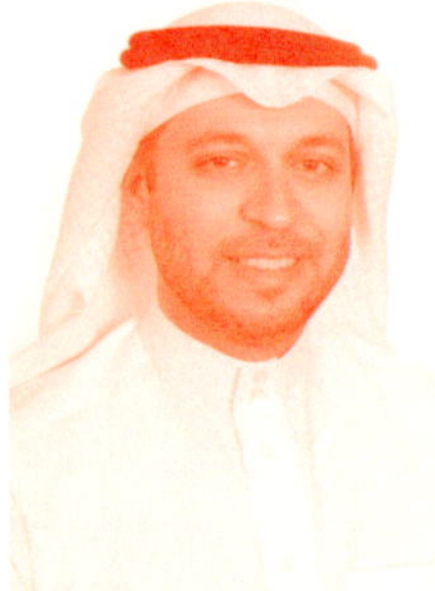
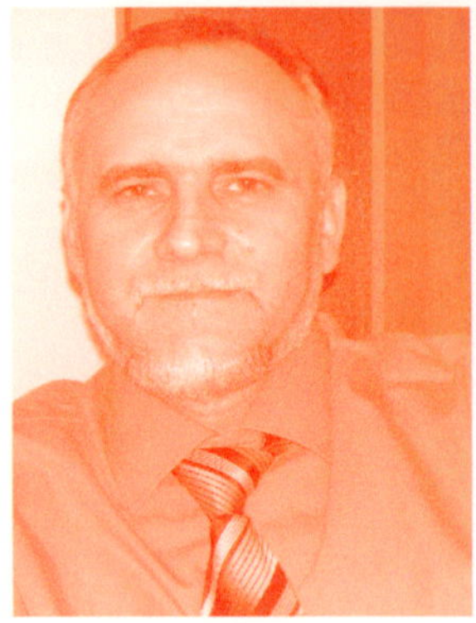
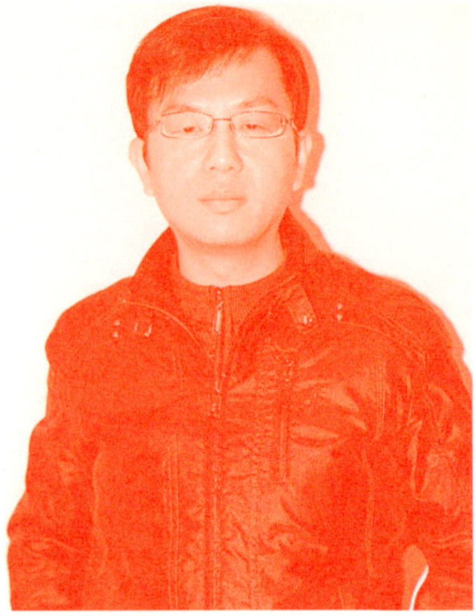
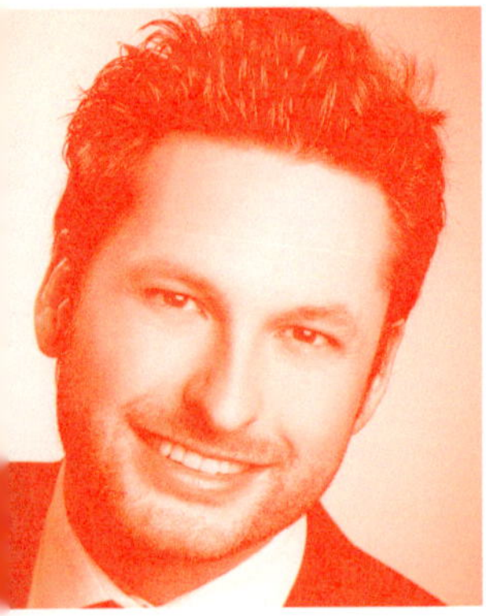
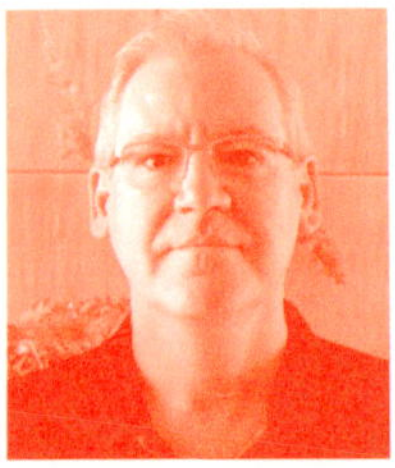

IntechOpen

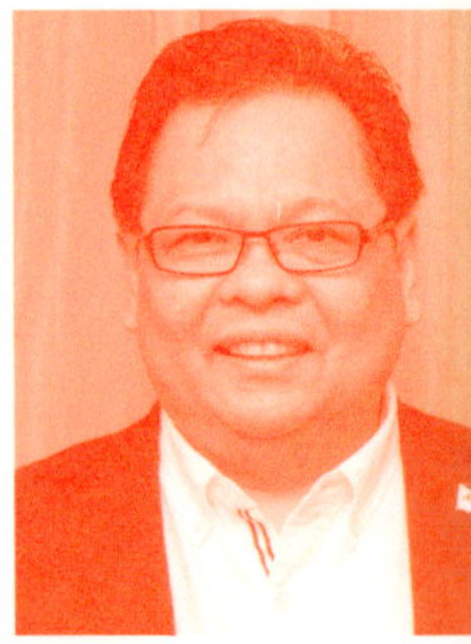
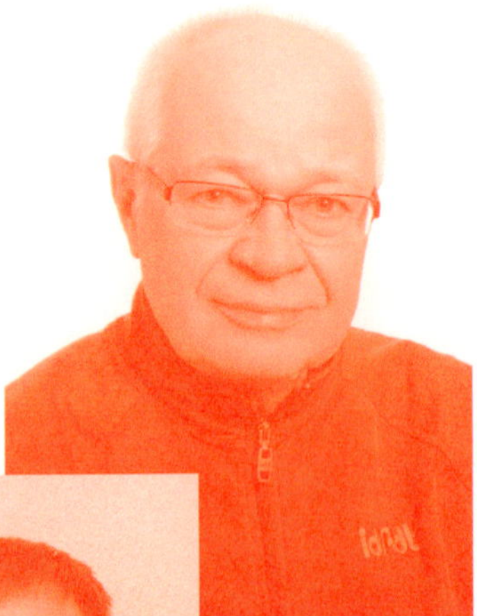
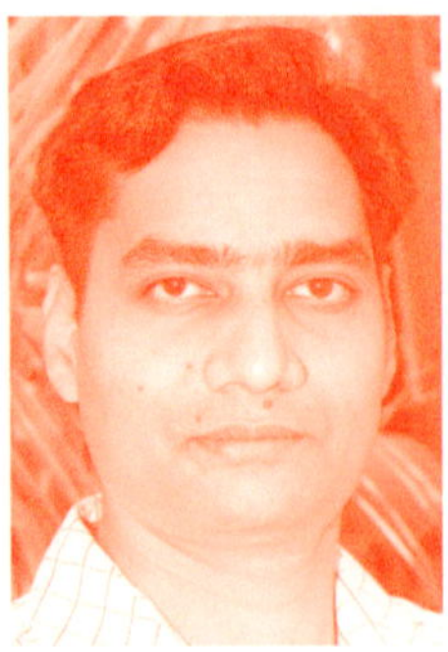
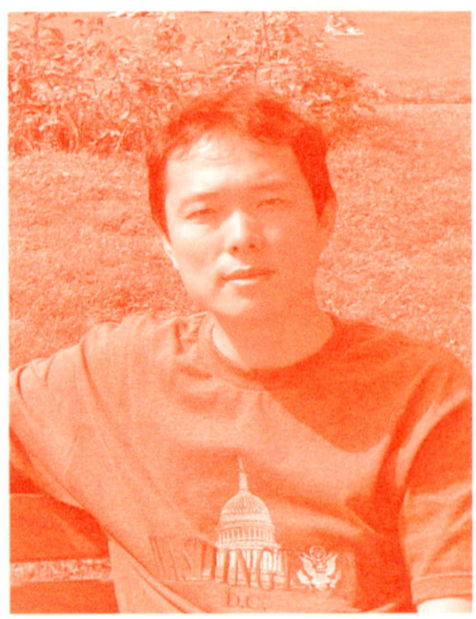
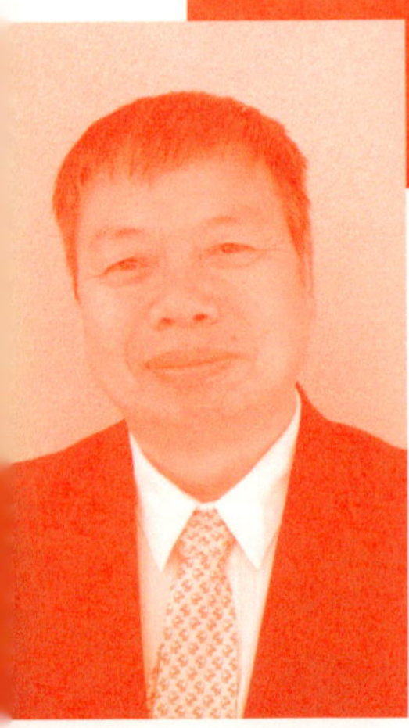
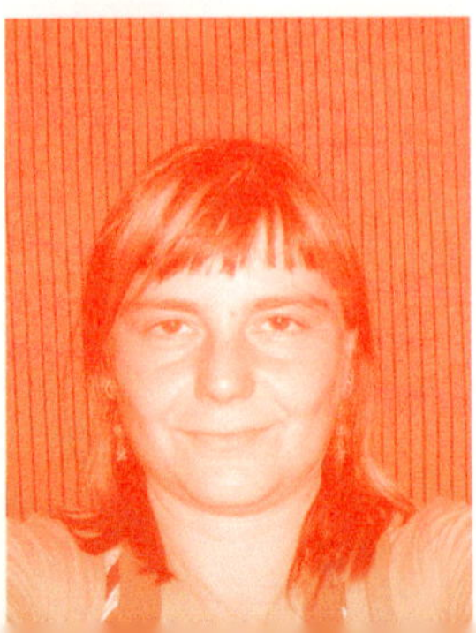

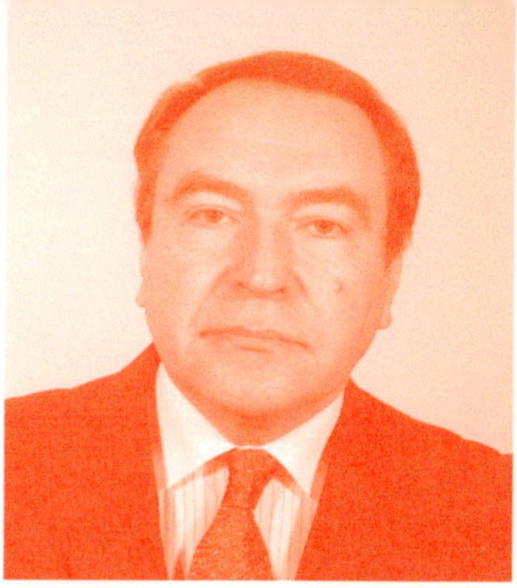
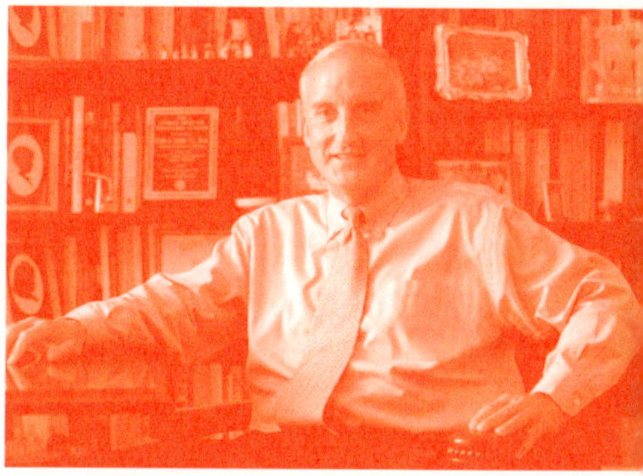
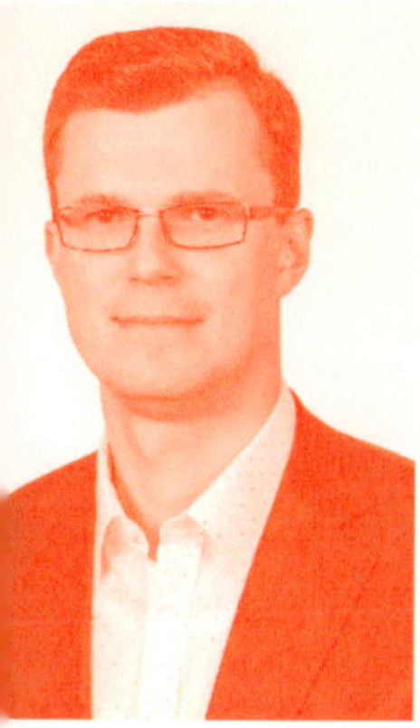
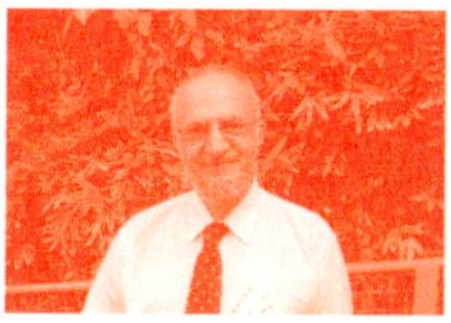
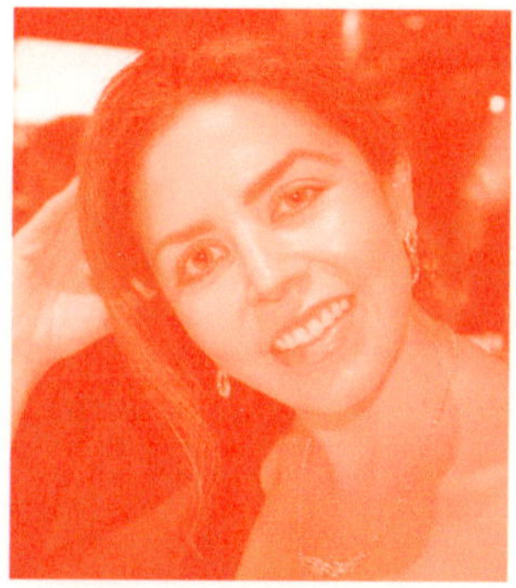

Supporting open minds since 2005

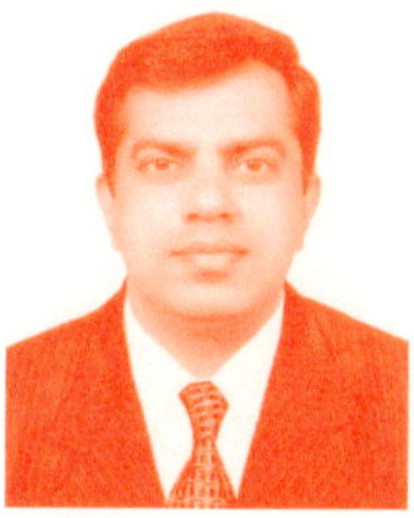
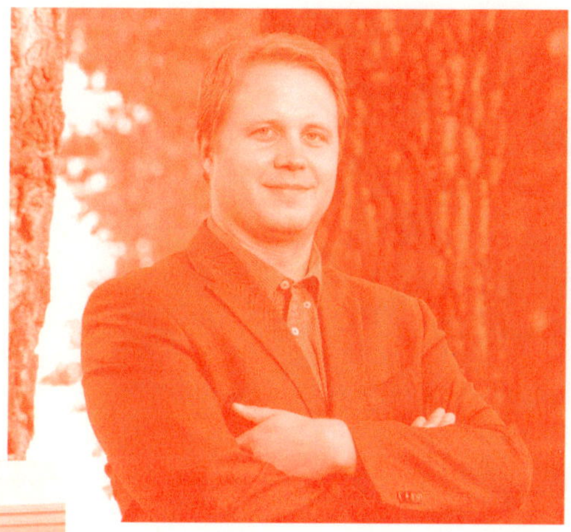
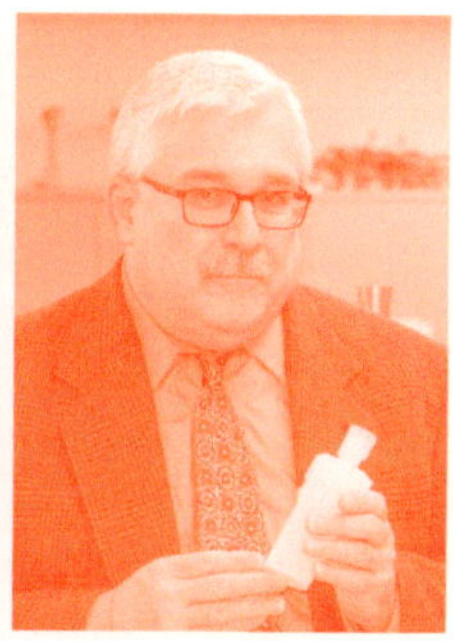
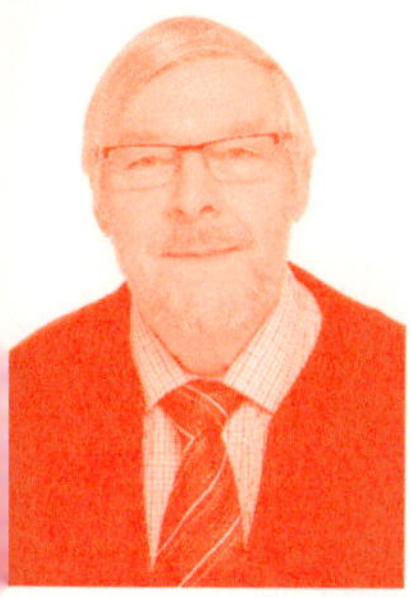
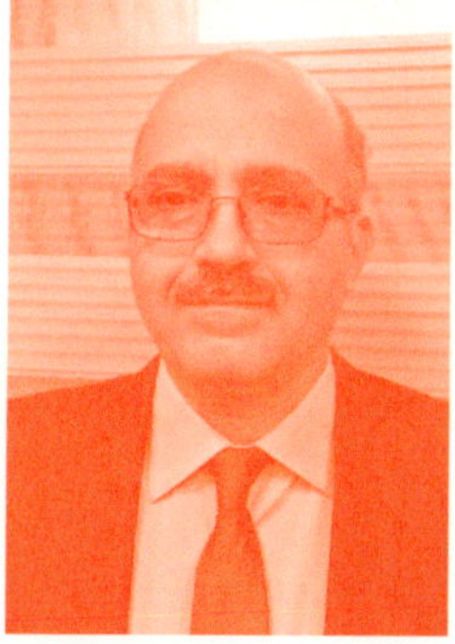
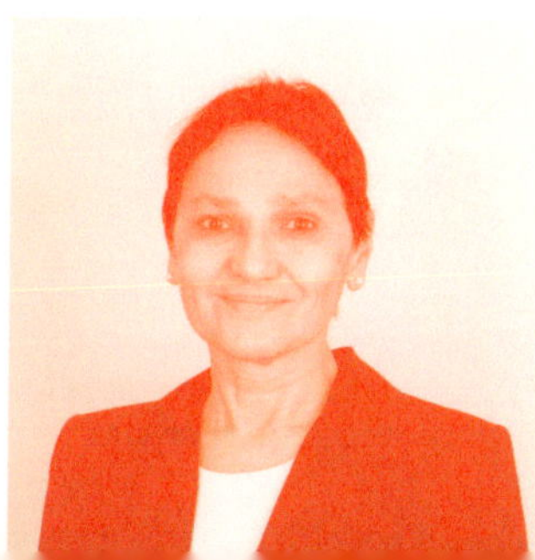
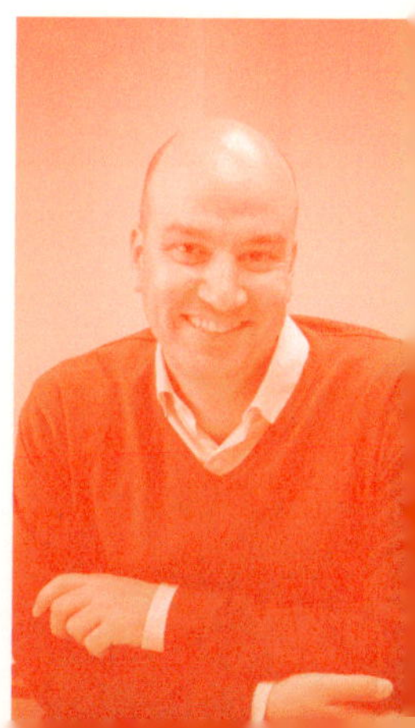

Recent Advances in Cesarean Delivery
http://dx.doi.org/10.5772/intechopen.78827
Edited by Georg Schmölzer

Contributors
Niamh Murphy, Naomi Burke, Fionnuala Breathnach, Constantin Zwergel, Constantin von Kaisenberg, Kristina Roloff, Guillermo Valenzuela, Suzanne Cao, Camille Okekpe, Inessa Dombrovsky, Josaphat Byamugisha, Moses Adroma, Satoru Takeda, Jun Takeda, Shintaro Makino, Ioannis Kosmas, Ospan Mynbaev, Zhongjie Shi, Avinoam Tzabari, Leila Kindarova, Styliani Salta, Lin Ma, Antonio Malvasi, Andrea Tinelli, Victor Gomel, Tatiana Babenko, Ivano Raimondo, Michael Stark

First published in London, United Kingdom, 2020 by IntechOpen
IntechOpen is the global imprint of INTECHOPEN LIMITED, registered in England and Wales, registration number: 11086078, 7th floor, 10 Lower Thames Street, London, EC3R 6AF, United Kingdom
Printed in Croatia

British Library Cataloguing-in-Publication Data
A catalogue record for this book is available from the British Library

Additional hard and PDF copies can be obtained from orders@intechopen.com

Recent Advances in Cesarean Delivery
Edited by Georg Schmölzer
p. cm.
Print ISBN 978-1-78984-694-2
Online ISBN 978-1-78984-695-9
eBook (PDF) ISBN 978-1-78984-205-0

For EU product safety concerns:
IN TECH d.o.o., Prolaz Marije Krucifikse Kozulić 3, 51000 Rijeka, Croatia, info@intechopen.com or visit our website at intechopen.com.

Meet the editor

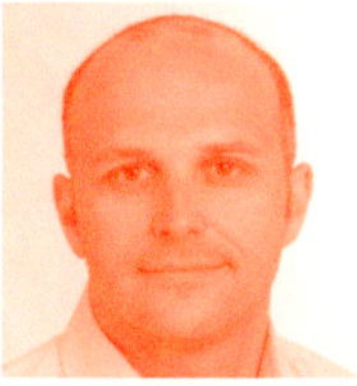

Dr. Schmölzer is the inaugural Heart and Stroke Foundation/ University of Alberta Professor of Neonatal Resuscitation and the Director of the Center for the Studies on Asphyxia and Resuscitation (CSAR) in Edmonton, Alberta, Canada. He also works as a neonatologist at the Royal Alexandra Hospital, Alberta, Canada. Dr. Schmölzer obtained an MD, PhD, and clinical training in Austria and Australia. In 2014, he completed a Banting Postdoctoral Fellowship at the University of Alberta. Dr. Schmölzer's research focuses on understanding physiological changes during fetal-to-neonatal transition, improving diagnoses, mitigating risk, and improving survival and quality of life for newborns, using emerging technologies during neonatal resuscitation, and examining how these physiological changes can be used to improve short- and long-term outcomes of newborn babies.

Contents

Preface

A cesarean section is a life-saving surgical procedure when certain complications arise during pregnancy and labor. *Recent Advances in Cesarean Delivery* is a collection of research chapters on cesarean delivery and related developments within the field of obstetrics. Written by experts in the field, chapters cover such topics as prediction of cesarean delivery, hemostasis for massive hemorrhage during C-section, maternal and fetal risks, cesarean scar defect manifestations, obesity and C-section, and C-sections in low-, middle-, and high-income countries.

IntechOpen

Chapter 1

Prediction of Caesarean Delivery

Niamh C. Murphy, Fionnuala M. Breathnach and Naomi Burke

Abstract

For expectant parents, a first birth is notable for its unpredictability, and the path to safe labour and delivery is commonly complicated by a requirement for unplanned caesarean delivery. The ability to anticipate an uncomplicated vaginal birth, or to predict the requirement for unplanned caesarean delivery, carries the potential to facilitate optimal birth choices. For example, elective caesarean delivery confers substantially less risk than unplanned caesarean delivery performed during the course of labour. Pre-delivery knowledge of a high predictive risk of requiring intrapartum caesarean delivery could lead to women opting to deliver by elective caesarean delivery, thereby lowering associated risks. Equally, pre-labour knowledge of a high prospect of achieving a successful and uncomplicated vaginal birth could result in enhanced motivation for women to deliver in a less medicalised environment. Predictive risk models have been utilised to good effect in other areas of medicine. The incorporation of a risk predictive tool for intrapartum caesarean delivery would enable women and their caregivers to choose the most appropriate management plan for each woman.

Keywords: prediction model, caesarean delivery, personalised care

1. Introduction

The last three decades have witnessed an escalation in global Caesarean section rates. It is well recognised that there is an association between delivery by Caesarean section and both short and long-term maternal morbidity, particularly at an advanced stage in labour [1]. This association is significantly stronger in the setting of emergency Caesarean section than scheduled elective non-labour Caesarean delivery.

It is notable that post-operative complications, including haemorrhage and perioperative infection in women who undergo unplanned Caesarean delivery are significantly higher when compared to women who undergo elective Caesarean delivery [2].

Magann et al. [3] examined the outcomes regarding post-partum haemorrhage of over 4000 Caesarean section deliveries in Australia in their observational study. They determined that the incidence of post-partum haemorrhage in an emergency setting was 6.75% and the incidence in an elective setting was 4.74%.

A 2014 Cochrane review [4] examined the rates of post-partum sepsis for both intrapartum and elective caesarean sections. They identified 95 studies, which recruited over 15,000 women. They determined that the rates of wound infection were 9.7 and 6.8% respectively. As regards endometritis, the rates were 18.4% for intrapartum caesarean sections versus 3.9% for elective caesarean sections.

It is important to also reference the association in particular between intrapartum caesarean sections and maternal morbidity. The incidence of caesarean sections performed at full dilatation is increasing [5]. These deliveries are associated with an increase in maternal morbidity including visceral trauma, haemorrhage and extension of the wound [6].

The Archives of Obstetrics and Gynaecology published a review in 2017 which specifically aimed to enumerate the differences in complications experienced in women who underwent elective Caesarean delivery and those who underwent emergency Caesarean delivery [7].

This systematic review included nine individual studies. Inclusion criteria dictated that the studies had to be either a randomised control trial study or a controlled clinical trial study to perform a comparison of the morbidity and mortality between elective and emergency intrapartum Caesarean delivery.

The combined results demonstrated that the rates of infection, fever, urinary tract infection, wound dehiscence, disseminated intravascular coagulopathy, and reoperation of emergency Caesarean section were all much higher than those of elective Caesarean section.

A unifying sentiment that can dominate a woman's post-natal course after an intrapartum Caesarean section delivery is the desire to anticipate this intervention. Prenatal knowledge that a successful vaginal birth will not be achieved would obviate the labour-associated risks that frequently result in maternal or perinatal morbidity, and the dissatisfaction of having undergone a 'trial' of labour to no avail.

The Organisation for Economic Co-Operation and Development (OECD) reports that there has been a significant increase in Caesarean section delivery rates in most OECD countries between the years 2000 and 2015. The average rate has increased from 20 to 28%, although there does appear to have been a slow-down in the rate of growth in the past 5 years [8]. It is also notable that different hospitals and regions within the same country can show significant variation in their Caesarean section rates. For example, Italy continues to show huge variation in the Caesarean delivery rates. High rates of Caesarean delivery appear to be driven by the southern region. Similar variations in rates between different regions are also observed in Spain [9].

Of note, the U.S. has shown a decline in its Caesarean delivery rate for the fourth consecutive year. Caesarean delivery rates in 2016 were 31.9%, which had fallen slightly from 32% in 2015. Prior to this, they had increased annually from 20.7% in 1996 to a peak of 32.95 in 2009 [10].

On a global level, the Caesarean section rate over the past 30 years has escalated but interestingly, no associated significant maternal or perinatal benefits have been demonstrated [11–13].

This increase prompted The Lancet to compile a series on optimising the use of Caesarean section, which was published in October 2018. The authors of this review argued that the decision to perform a Caesarean section might be guided by the psychological or clinical needs of the mother, the clinical needs of the baby or by a combination of both [14].

However, where rates of Caesarean section exceed what is considered a 'recommended rate' of 10–15% as per the World Health Organisation [15], there were three main drivers identified which were though to contribute to perceived over-use of this intervention. These were categorised broadly as health professionals; communities (incorporating families, childbearing women and the broader society) and health care systems (comprising organisational design and cultures and financing).

As regards communities, families, childbearing women and the broader society, it was noted that women worldwide would not prefer to have a Caesarean section without a significant maternal or foetal indication [16]. This is in direct contrast to the common perception that many women would choose a Caesarean section as a matter of preference [17].

Factors relating to health professionals highlighted that being male, being employed in a university-affiliated hospital and a fear of litigation were associated with an increased likelihood of an obstetrician performing a Caesarean section [14]. They also found Caesarean section might sometimes be used for convenience. This was particularly noted where both a combination of private and public work was performed in the same unit. The scheduling of elective Caesarean sections can allow commitments to public work being fulfilled while allowing the performance of private work on the same premises [18].

Of particular interest to clinicians is addressing the safe prevention of unwarranted primary Caesarean section delivery. In March 2014, a joint consensus was issued by the Society for Maternal Fetal Medicine and American College of Obstetricians and Gynaecologists (ACOG). This addressed the importance of the safe prevention of primary Caesarean delivery and this was reaffirmed in 2016 [19]. As previously mentioned, The Lancet has also highlighted the importance of addressing appropriate and safe use of Caesarean section in order to address the escalating rates worldwide [9].

This chapter will deal with the use of prediction models in medicine in order to address how best to antenatally predict the need for an intrapartum Caesarean section for a nulliparous woman. The clinical application of such a prediction model would ultimately be that those women issued with a high likelihood for intrapartum Caesarean delivery might opt for an elective Caesarean section with the associated decreased morbidity risks.

On a corollary to this is the point that many women would likely prefer the prospect of a trial of labour if they were assigned a low-risk for intrapartum caesarean delivery. Furthermore, this may allow women the opportunity to consider a less medicalised environment for birth for example in a midwifery-led unit. A review of the literature would suggest that the majority of women would opt for a vaginal delivery over a caesarean section. An Australian study which asked women to complete an antenatal questionnaire found that 93.5% of women would prefer a vaginal delivery over a caesarean section [20]. This showed very similar results to a Swedish-based study which found that only 8.2% of nulliparous women would prefer to deliver by caesarean section [21]. Similar opinions were also found amongst women in Brazil and Chile, which are countries with traditionally high caesarean section rates [22–24]. The Genesis risk prediction model could empower women entering labour with a low predictive risk score for an intrapartum caesarean section that they had a high likelihood of a desirable successful vaginal delivery.

I will outline the development and usage of prediction models in other areas of medicine and the research into various factors, which have been highlighted as predictive for Caesarean delivery. If achievable, the ability to predict the outcome of an attempt at first labour is highly desirable. It is apparent that the safe prevention of primary Caesarean delivery is an outcome, which would be welcomed by the international obstetric community.

2. Predictive models

2.1 Rationale for use of predictive models in healthcare

Certain decisions in healthcare require a detailed process in order to provide optimal care to patients. This can be complicated by a deficit in standardisation of processes, which aim to encompass the needs of multiple stakeholders.

Various modelling tools can assist the decision-making process. Some of these aim to predict a clinical outcome, whereas others focus on identifying the patients who may be most at risk of developing a certain condition [25].

These tools are created using formulae that may assist in decision-making. These in turn can assist in resource planning and allocation in healthcare. Examples of such tools are prognostic and prediction models [26].

Prognostic models may have varied uses, including 'guiding healthcare policy by generating global prediction scenarios; determining study eligibility of patients for new treatments; selecting appropriate tests and therapies in individual patient management including supporting decisions on withholding or withdrawing therapy' [27].

The two main types of prognostic models seen in practice are those at the individual patient level and those at the patient population level. Individual patient models are used in suggesting advice for treatment and to provide consultation, which is patient-centered. Patient population models are more focused on the identification of discrepancies and trends amongst patient groups for a specific criterion [27].

Predictive modelling can be used to help identity patients who may be at high-risk for a certain outcome, e.g. an intrapartum Caesarean delivery. Predictive modelling can also be used in order to manage healthcare resources by initiating appropriate interventions to prevent high-cost outcomes [28].

One such example which has been developed in clinical practice is the cardiovascular disease risk assessment for primary prevention. The Framingham Heart Study looked at 7733 participants who had initially been free of coronary heart disease and were aged between 40 and 79 years. They found that the lifetime risk of being affected by coronary heart disease (CHD) for these participants by age 40 was 32% in women and 49% in men [29].

This highlighted the importance of cardiovascular disease risk assessment being performed from the age of 20 years of age or from a person's first encounter with the healthcare system. This can then in turn predict those individuals who are at the most significant risk of cardiovascular disease. Identifiable risk factors included cigarette smoking, hypertension, diabetes mellitus, premature family history of cardiovascular disease, chronic kidney disease and obesity. These individuals can then be commenced on appropriate primary preventive therapies or receive alternative appropriate intervention. Predictive modelling acts on the basis of taking a proactive approach, i.e. the identification of trends and forecasting of events which may cause implications for stakeholders in healthcare [25].

There are several factors which need to be considered in the implementation of a new prediction model [30]. These include:

- The creation of a focus on the population as a whole and examining all aspects of healthcare
- An emphasis on change of behaviour in the longer-term
- The utilisation of data to create programs which aim to address learning, health status and individualised risk
- The development of health plan designs which act to support and incentivise

Providers of healthcare and patients are both motivated to achieve improved outcomes and this suggests that the use of these models is likely to increase with the added benefit of potential reduction in healthcare costs.

For our purposes, accurate prediction of Caesarean delivery may allow consideration being given to elective Caesarean delivery in the event of a woman being considered high risk for an intrapartum Caesarean delivery in order to reduce the incidence of specific maternal morbidities as aforementioned including infection, haemorrhage and the need for a repeat surgery. A low predictive risk score also empowers women who are keen on a successful vaginal delivery with the knowledge that they have a high likelihood of achieving same.

2.2 Use of predictive models in obstetrics

Historically, the field of obstetrics has been successful in developing prediction models but has been poor in fully validating and thus implementing them effectively [31].

On a daily basis, we still use two examples of prognostic models in obstetrics, which were developed over 60 years ago. One such model is the Apgar score, which assesses newborn babies immediately after their birth. The other model is the Bishop score, which assesses the status of the cervix before and during induction of labour [32, 33]. Both of these models were developed in the 1950s–1960s and are still used clinically, likely due to their ease of use and continued relevance [31].

The Apgar score was re-examined and re-validated by a research group in Texas almost 50 years after its initial introduction. They reviewed the charts of more than 150,000 deliveries over a 10 years period and found there was a significant correlation between these babies' 5 minute Apgar scores and neonatal mortality [34]. This score remains an easy and quick way to determine if resuscitation has been effective and has therefore survived the test of time [35].

The Bishop score assesses cervical dilatation, cervical effacement, cervical consistency, cervical position and foetal station. A higher score meant a woman was more likely to have a spontaneous onset of labour sooner. It is still in use today and can aid clinicians in deciding the most appropriate method of delivery for each woman. The work of Professors Apgar and Bishop essentially formed some of our earliest prediction models in obstetrics.

Only two thirds of the papers [62.4%, 164/263] in a large systematic review of prognostic models in obstetrics were found to have presented their models in such a way that external validation would be feasible [31]. This has been highlighted as a concern given the importance of validity in the development of such models.

Certain models can be too complex for routine clinical usage and this may lead to a reluctance on the part of the clinicians to accept them [36]. For example, the use of an electronic program to help predict those patients most in need of requiring an influenza vaccination was found to be ineffective as it did not prove to be user-friendly. It is also important that models which have been developed are also validated in a new population as otherwise it may not be possible to generalise them to a different cohort of patients [37]. This is also known as impact analysis and this paper by Reilly et al. highlights that very few prediction models have undergone formal impact analysis or validation. This is essential in order for clinicians to know if the usage of such a model will have a positive or negative effect, i.e. is there a possibility that it will cause harm. The authors highlighted the benefit of having clinicians involved in the development and validation of such models before, during and after implementation.

There are limitations to the development and use of prediction models in obstetrics. It has been shown that internal validation is largely successful and the models have been shown to perform well under this setting. However, there has been a deficit of research into looking in to externally validating these prediction models in a different cohort. Another limiting factor for clinical usage and which was discussed in a commentary in the British Journal of Obstetrics and Gynaecology (BJOG) in 2016 is how interventions might be handled in a prediction model [38]. This commentary highlighted the issues, which face clinicians in validating obstetric prediction models in order to effectively implement them in clinical practice. They specifically examined the area of pre-eclampsia and noted that a phenomenon described as the treatment paradox can occur; a strong predictor of a common complication may trigger an effective treatment (e.g. commencement of anti-hypertensive therapy) at an early stage and this will then prevent the occurrence of a certain proportion of adverse outcomes. This may result in the predictor, which triggered the treatment initially appearing poorer in its predictive performance [39, 40].

The BJOG review [38] further examined a prediction model which has been successfully validated for the predicting pre-eclampsia (PREP model-Development and validation of Prediction models for Risks of complications in Early-onset Pre-eclampsia) [41] in order to ascertain what made it a successful process and highlighted certain factors which can aid validation. These included large sample size, standardisation of treatment or intervention, and the consideration to the initiation of treatment being an outcome itself, i.e. 'When starting a treatment is likely to prevent an adverse outcome, those who received the treatment could also be considered to have experienced the outcome'. These factors may aid obstetricians in validation of prediction models going forward and in handling the treatment paradox.

2.3 Use of predictive models in gynaecology

The field of gynaecology has also developed a new risk prediction model in recent times. A large cross-sectional international cohort study involved the participation of 5020 patients from 22 centres [42]. This study developed and validated a risk prediction model to predict the risk of malignancy in adnexal masses using specific ultrasound features which are defined in the simple rules.

In 2008, the simple rules were described by the International Ovarian Tumour Analysis (IOTA) group [43]. These specific ultrasound features are known as either B-features (where tumours are likely benign) or M-features (where tumours are likely malignant).

In using the simple rules, and there are no specific features identified or if there is a conflict between the features, then the rules cannot be applied and the result is inconclusive. In this instance, it is recommended to classify the findings as having a higher risk of malignancy in order to increase the sensitivity for ovarian cancer [33].

The simple rules have been well received by clinicians and adopted by international bodies such as the Royal College of Obstetricians and Gynaecologists [34]. Zimmerman et al. aimed to develop and validate a model based on the criteria laid down in the simple rules. When used as originally suggested, the simple rules aimed to categorise tumours as belonging to one of three distinct groups: benign, malignant, or inconclusive. Zimmerman et al. demonstrated that the simple rules could also be used to estimate the risk of malignancy in every adnexal mass. In this way, they can be applied to individual patients to optimise their own management [31]. The rules were found to be applicable in 76% (386/507) of the tumours, with a sensitivity of 95% (106/112) and a specificity of 91% (249/274). This risk prediction model has the potential to be broadly accepted given its ease of use and the fact that it is based on standards which have already been accepted and are used by the gynaecological community. Several follow up studies [35, 36] have highlighted that the rules can be easily utilised by ultrasonographers and that the protocol can be an accurate test to diagnose ovarian cancer.

2.4 Use of predictive models in other aspects of health care

Increasingly, attempts have been made to develop and validate prediction tools which aim to predict the risk of hospital readmission [44]. Interest in this area has evolved for a number of reasons. Of clinical importance is that an intervention while a patient remains in hospital may help to reduce readmission rates as those in need of additional care may receive it while still an inpatient. It also helps to target delivery of interventions which are resource-intensive to those with the greatest need [45]. This would result in a stratification of the risk of readmission, which may hold clinical relevance. In turn, this would allow for early information during a patient's admission, which would allow the initiation of an intervention such as advanced discharge planning which could begin during the admission and before discharge from hospital. Models used should be accurate, clinically relevant, use easily obtainable data and be able to be used in large patient populations [46].

Covariates are used in risk prediction models. This is done with the aim of detecting a given outcome or to determine a defined period of time whereby an individual is thought to experience a specific outcome [47].

These predictors are varied and may encompass characteristics such as gender or age, biochemical markers, coronary artery deposits or specific genetic markers [48].

In the field of cardiology, prediction models include Framingham [49], SCORE [50], ASSIGN [51], EUROSCORE [52], PROCAM [53], and Wells' scores [54].

Prediction models may assist individuals and their clinicians in deciding the most appropriate management plan or on the implementation or withholding of treatment or lifestyle interventions.

There is an increased desire to implement personalised care and because of this, research into prediction models is increasing [55]. In the current era of risk-tailored and personalised cardiovascular care, studies on prediction models are abundant. A recent statement of the American Heart Association on criteria for the phased evaluation of markers of cardiovascular risk underlines this. A key term in this statement was that 'multivariable prediction models and cardiovascular markers should not (simply) be evaluated in isolation for their prediction abilities but rather on their added prediction contribution beyond existing or established predictors requiring a multivariable approach in design, conduct, analyses and reporting' [56].

It is important that the development of prediction models should follow strict methodologic processes. New prediction models should detail their development process and highlight all their statistical calculations in order to allow researchers in the future to reproduce and validate their findings. Research into the relatively new field of biomarkers needs to determine their additional benefit to pre-existing models [57].

The selection of specific chemotherapy regimens is made based on examination of the outcomes for specific subtypes and specific types of malignant tumours, their likelihood to progress to metastases and their overall prognosis [58, 59]. The overall effectiveness of certain agents also means that the development of tiered strategies has developed in order to overcome variations seen in the resistance of certain tumours [60].

This study examined the responses of chemotherapy agents cisplatin, carboplatin and oxaliplatin with certain gene signatures [61]. This group developed a machine-learning based prediction model, which aimed to predict the effectiveness of the agents above to certain gene signatures. This tailored treatment may result in an improved treatment response to an individual's specific cancer biology which may result in reduced treatment duration or the minimum usage of chemotherapy agents to achieve a desired response [62].

Cancer treatment is challenging as the disease can be complicated by genetic heterogeneity with differences in the genetic composition of tumours causing different responses to treatment [63].

The impact of this variance in genetic composition means that there may varied responses to treatment regimes. This means that the therapy may only benefit a small proportion of the patients treated [64]. In order to minimise the associated adverse effects which can occur with using these treatments, it is of particular benefit to patients with cancer to decide on the optimal treatment regime at the time of diagnosis [65].

Ubels et al. [65] developed the idea of simulated treatment learning (STL). This program assists in identifying the factors that can best predict treatment benefit and can be applied to gene expression datasets with two treatment arms and associated survival data. It works by identifying genetic similarities between patients from different groups to model how a particular patient would respond to an alternative treatment plan and is defined based on the expression of the genes in the tumour. Their work focused on patients with multiple myeloma and how best to predict the benefit of treatment. Multiple myeloma affects the bone marrow by causing abnormal multiplication of the plasma cells. The typical median survival is approximately 5 years [66]. Multiple myeloma is one of the known conditions where a difference in gene expression profiles is observed amongst patients [67]. This variation in genes expression means that identification of individual genetic signatures may be useful to help predict those who would benefit from STL.

3. Prediction of intrapartum caesarean section

3.1 Definition of intrapartum caesarean section

An intrapartum Caesarean section is a Caesarean section, which occurs during the course of labour. According to the American College of Obstetricians and Gynaecology, the most common indications for primary Caesarean delivery include, in order of frequency, labour dystocia, abnormal foetal heart rate tracing, foetal malpresentation, multiple gestation, and suspected foetal macrosomia [19].

3.2 Labour dystocia and associated risk factors

The progression of labour and recognition of prolonged labour can heavily influence the management of labour and the need for intrapartum Caesarean section. Prolonged labour has been defined as true labour dystocia and may be caused by either obstruction of labour or contractions, which are inadequate in number or strength. Prolonged labour is the main indication for performing an intrapartum Caesarean section in nulliparous patients [68].

Labour dystocia may be recognised in either the first or the second stage of labour. It has been reported to affect 21–37% of nulliparous women and 2–8% of multiparous women [69–71]. It has been attributed to several factors including macrosomia, reduced capacity of the pelvis, inefficient uterine contractions or a combination of these factors [72]. There are multiple studies in the literature examining the causes of labour dystocia.

The association between foetal macrosomia and labour dystocia is well described. Galvin et al. have previously looked at the accuracy of antenatal detection of macrosomia >4000 g and subsequent delivery outcomes in the absence of antenatal intervention [73]. They noted ultrasound sensitivity and specificity of 41.2 and 94.1% respectively for detecting macrosomia >4000 g. The positive predictive value (PPV) and negative predictive value (NPV) were 57.5 and 89.1% respectively. Their conclusion was that the capacity of ultrasound to detect foetal macrosomia is limited.

This finding is also reflected in a study by Chuahan et al. [74]. This group conducted a review of international articles from studies containing a sample size of at least 1000 cases in order to determine the prevalence and accuracy of determining macrosomia. The probability of detecting a macrosomic baby in a term, low-risk baby is ranged from 15 to 79% sonographically and 40–52% with clinical examination. They determined that the detection of macrosomia is reliable sonographically and clinically if the incidence of macrosomia is at least 20% in the relevant cohort.

The influence of foetal head circumference on delivery outcome has been extensively studied. Kennelly et al. suggested in 2003 that foetal head circumference >37 cm is a good predictor of prolonged labour in their study which examined 423 nulliparous women with a singleton cephalic presentation who had a spontaneous onset of labour [75]. They determined that as birth weight and foetal head circumference increased, there was an associated increase in mean duration of labour, duration of second stage of labour and usage of oxytocin ($P < 0.001$).

Elvander et al. conducted a population based register study, which was published in 2011 [76]. This examined a total of 265,456 singleton term neonates who were born to nulliparous women between 1999 and 2008 in Sweden. This data was extrapolated following analysis of the Swedish Medical Birth Register. The investigators examined factors including labour dystocia, instrumental delivery, foetal distress and Caesarean section. They found that the prevalence of each outcome increased as the circumference of the foetal head increased. In the case of Caesarean section in particular, the odds ratio was 1.22 (95% CI 1.04–1.42), indicating that a large foetal head (39–41 cm) is associated with labour dystocia and subsequent intrapartum Caesarean section. Valsky et al. also highlighted prolonged second stage of labour (greater than 110 minutes) and increasing foetal head circumference as risk factors for obstetric anal sphincter injury in nulliparous women. They showed through logistic regression that a head circumference greater than 35.5 cm and a second stage of labour greater than 110 minutes increased the odds of obstetric anal sphincter injury by a factor of 5.32 [77].

The position of the foetal head has also been extensively examined as a risk factor for Caesarean section. Occipito-posterior position is identified in approximately 15–20% of women before labour at term [78, 79]. The majority 90–95% undergo rotation during labour to an occipito-anterior position [80, 81]. The presence of an occipito-posterior position at delivery has been extensively examined with respect to maternal morbidity and an increased risk for Caesarean delivery [82–85].

Maternal age has been strongly associated with delivery by Caesarean section. Women aged 40 and over are more than twice as likely to deliver by Caesarean as women under age 20 [8]. Advanced maternal age has been shown to be associated with an increased risk of obesity [86], diabetes and hypertensive disease [87–89] and interventions including delivery by Caesarean section [90–94]. There is evidence demonstrating that the rate of Caesarean sections performed on an elective basis in the absence of a strong medical indication increases with advancing maternal age [95, 96]. Maternal age has also been shown to be an independent risk factor for Caesarean delivery [97].

Maternal BMI has also been associated with delivery by Caesarean section. Young and Woodmansee in 2003 published the results of an 8-year review of women who delivered in their practice. They found that primiparous woman who had a BMI of over $>30\ kg/m^2$ were six times more likely to undergo an intrapartum Caesarean delivery for labour dystocia than those primiparous women whose BMI was $<20\ kg/m^2$. This difference in mode of delivery persisted even when results were controlled for gestational age, birth weight, maternal height and maternal age [98].

Algovik et al. performed a retrospective analysis of the Swedish Birth Registry and identified 104 women in 47 families where at least two of sisters had undergone intrapartum Caesarean delivery at term attributed to labour dystocia during the course of a first labour [72]. A genetic basis for labour dystocia was sought, which identified strong evidence of linkage at chromosome 12p12 and at five other separate loci, which may of significance. There was no specific prevalence data included in their report. The authors however were unable to identify a specific gene, which may be responsible for labour dystocia. Re-sequencing of oxytocin (OXT) and oxytocin receptor (OXTR) seemed to be obvious candidate genes for this analysis. However, they did not allow for identification of any potential causal mutations. Further studies with a larger study population were recommended.

Mittal et al. [99] have also performed genetic testing to establish a cause for arrest of labour. They obtained myometrium samples from 50 women who underwent primary Caesarean delivery in a prospective study. All of these women had had a spontaneous onset of labour. They compared two groups of women. One group (n = 29) underwent Caesarean delivery due to either non-reassuring foetal status or foetal malpresentation. The second group (n = 21) underwent Caesarean delivery due to an arrest of labour. This was defined as women who had complete cervical dilatation but without continued foetal descent for greater than 1 hour. They identified over 400 different genes, which differed in women who experience an arrest in the descent of the foetal head during labour when compared with those who underwent Caesarean delivery for non-reassuring foetal status or foetal malpresentation. An over expression of certain inflammatory and biomarkers was identified in women who experience an arrest of descent including hypoxia inducible factor-1a, prostaglandin-endoperoxidase synthase 2 and interleukin-6. These factors were identified using micro-array. The authors did acknowledge that their study may be limited, as they could not establish a true causative effect, as this would require studies involving serial sampling in women, which would not be feasible. However, they recommended that this study may act as a framework for additional studies, which may address potential therapeutic interventions.

3.3 Model of care as a predictor of caesarean section rates

In many maternity settings worldwide, women can opt for obstetric or midwifery-led care. A descriptive comparative Australian study examined the outcomes of women who opted for either midwifery-led care or standard hospital care, which incorporated more input from the obstetric team. The study found that more women who opted for midwifery-led care were very satisfied with their overall care during their pregnancy, labour and delivery than those who experienced standard hospital care (80% very satisfied versus 53.2%). However, the study found that there was no observable difference in the Caesarean delivery rate between the two groups [100].

A randomised controlled trial, also based in Australia, examined if there was a difference in the Caesarean delivery rate between women who were assigned standard hospital-based care or community led care. However, this study differed from the aforementioned descriptive study in that those who experienced community led care were under the joint collaborative care of both midwives and obstetricians. In this study, there was a significant difference in the Caesarean delivery rate between the two groups. The group that experienced community based care had a Caesarean section rate of 13.3% (73/550) and the group that had standard hospital based care had a Caesarean section rate of 17.8% (96/539). The difference remained after controls were implemented for other known factors which may have contributed to their Caesarean sections (OR = 0.6, 95% CI 0.4–0.9, P = 0.02) [101].

A Canadian randomised controlled trial in 1996 examined the outcomes of nearly 200 low-risk women who were assigned randomly to either nurse-midwife led care or physician (family doctor and obstetrician) led care. The nurse-midwife led group had a Caesarean deliver rate of 4% in comparison with 15.1% in the physician group. There were also lower rates of epidural and episiotomy usage in the nurse-midwife led group [102].

Their relatively low numbers may explain the variations in the reported findings of these studies. The British Journal of Obstetrics and Gynaecology performed a systematic review in 2005 of randomised controlled trials in which the study intervention was characterised as midwifery-led care versus standard obstetric care. This review highlighted seven trials, including 9148 women. In general, they found that women who experienced midwifery-led care in their antenatal and labour courses were less likely to have interventions in labour including induction of labour, use of oxytocin, epidural usage, CTG monitoring, operative vaginal delivery and episiotomy. However there was no difference in the Caesarean delivery rate between the two groups (OR 0.91; 95% CI 0.78–1.05) and there were no observable differences in infant and maternal outcomes. [103].

The British Journal of Obstetrics and Gynaecology published the 'Birthplace study' in 2011 [104]. This large prospective cohort-based study of 64,538 women had the objective of comparing perinatal outcomes, maternal outcomes and interventions in labour by planned place of birth at the start of care in labour for women with low risk pregnancies. This study took place in NHS care facilities across England. Recruitment criteria included both nulliparous and multiparous women. The Birthplace study concluded that a choice of birth setting was optimal for women with low risk pregnancies and determined that those women who delivered in a midwifery unit or multiparous women who delivered at home experienced fewer interventions with no change in perinatal outcomes. When specifically comparing intrapartum Caesarean section rates, intended place of birth (with this decision made antenatally) varied significantly. Those who intended to give birth in an obstetric unit had an intrapartum Caesarean section rate of 11.1% (99% CI 9.5–13.0). This compared with those who intended to give birth in a midwifery unit or at home having intrapartum caesarean delivery rates of 3.5% (99% CI 2.8–4.2) and 2.8% (99% CI 2.3–3.4) respectively.

3.4 External pelvimetry

It is estimated that 600,000 worldwide die annually as a result of complications of pregnancy [105]. Of these, approximately 25% are thought to be attributable to cephalo-pelvic disproportion [105–108]. Cephalopelvic disproportion is defined as a mismatch between the size of the foetal head and size of the maternal pelvis, resulting in 'failure to progress' in labour for mechanical reasons [109]. It is therefore of significant global public health benefit to be able to accurately predict and detect these women who are more likely to require Caesarean section and to be in a position to predict this prior to labour onset. This is of particular importance in areas where Caesarean section is not feasible in order to be able to refer these women to units where Caesarean section may be performed. In the developed world where access to Caesarean section is easier, it is also desirable to be in a position to accurately predict those women who may require same, thus the importance of development of prediction models for Caesarean section.

External pelvimetry was the first known technique used to predict cephalopelvic disproportion [110, 111]. It involves the usage of a pelvimeter (e.g. Breisky pelvimeter). August Briesky was an Austrian gynaecologist who developed a pelvimeter in the nineteenth century in order to aim to accurately measure the dimensions of the female pelvis. A prospective cohort study published in the British Journal of Obstetrics and Gynaecology in 2000 by Liselele et al. [110] outlined the findings of 605 nulliparous women carried out in four hospitals in Zaire. They assessed maternal height and pelvimetry at the third trimester antenatal visit in order to predict women at risk for cephalo-pelvic disproportion with subsequent increased risk of Caesarean section. They considered women with a height less than 150 cm and/or external pelvic distances less than the 10th centile (<9.5 cm) for the population to be at highest risk. A height gauge was used to ascertain maternal height and pelvimetry was assessed externally using a Breisky pelvimeter. They considered cephalopelvic disproportion to be present in 42 women. Their analysis showed that maternal height less than 150 cm and/or transverse diagonal of the Michaelis sacral rhomboid area less than 9.5 cm were most likely to be associated with cephalopelvic disproportion and labour dystocia (odds ratio of 2.2 [95% CI 0.9–5.4] and 6.5 [95% CI 3.2–13.2], respectively]. They also showed a positive predictive value of 24% [95% CI 2–8 to 5–8]) [110]. The transverse diagonal of the Michaelis sacral rhomboid area assessed by pelvimetry was noted to be of significant importance in the development of a model. The authors of this study recommended external validation of this model in a separate cohort before it becomes implemented in clinical practice. With a PPV of 24% this did not translate into a worthy research pursuit in high resource income setting. However, it is worth considering in the low resource setting where timely access to skilled birth attendants may be considerably restricted.

In 2007, Rozenholc et al. [112] performed another prospective cohort study specifically incorporating the measurement of the transverse diagonal of the Michaelis sacral rhomboid area which had been noted to be predictive by Liselele et al. previously, along with other anthropometic measurements including maternal height. This study looked at 807 nulliparous term women at term who completed a trial of labour and delivered a singleton fetus with a cephalic presentation. Ninety-eight women (12.1%) were found to have labour dystocia. They concluded the combination of the maternal height with the transverse diagonal of the Michaelis sacral rhomboid area could identify, before labour, more than half of the cases of dystocia in nulliparous women, therefore being a useful prediction model for prediction of Caesarean section.

3.5 X-ray pelvimetry

X-ray can also be used to assess pelvimetry. This is usually done by measuring the pelvic outlet, pelvic inlet and mid-pelvis using conventional x-rays with an anterior-posterior and a lateral view [113]. A Cochrane review published in 2017 identified a total of 1159 women who had participated in five separate trials. All five of these trials used X-ray pelvimetry in pregnancy [114]. This review found that there was insufficient evidence to support the routine use of X-ray pelvimetry for assisting with decision making in determining the most appropriate mode of delivery for women. They concluded that women who underwent an X-ray pelvimetry may have an increased likelihood of undergoing a Caesarean section without any improved benefits for the woman or baby.

3.6 MRI pelvimetry

The usage of MRI has now been applied to pelvimetry. This has potential advantages including the fact that there is no exposure of mother or fetus to radiation and the higher calibre of the quality of images makes it easier to calculate the volume of the maternal pelvis and the foetal head [115].

Sporri et al. in their prospective observational study published in 2002 also determined that the efficacy of MRI for clinical use in dystocia is limited and recommended further research in order to determine the most appreciate anatomical landmarks which should be examined [116].

In 2004, Zaretsky et al. published their findings on MRI assessment of pelvimetry and its usage in the prediction of labour dystocia in another prospective study. This involved performing an MRI on 101 nulliparous women who were scheduled for an induction of labour for post-term pregnancy (>42 weeks). They found that MRI is accurate at predicting women who are at significant risk for labour dystocia but it is not of significant benefit when compared with other methods of pelvimetry [117].

3.7 Models for predicting vaginal birth after caesarean section

There is a significant body of research, which has examined the ability to predict a successful vaginal birth after a previous Caesarean section (VBAC).

The National institute of Child Health and Human Development Maternal-Fetal Medicine Units Network created a registry between 1999 and 2002 that incorporated the pregnancy outcomes of women who delivered at their 19 units. Using this data, a prediction model was developed to provide individual risk of probability of a successful VBAC for women with a singleton, cephalic presentation fetus at term who had experienced one prior Caesarean section. The data of 11,856 women were analysed. The key predictors include maternal BMI, maternal age, body mass index, ethnicity (Caucasian women having higher success rates), timing of the vaginal delivery in relation to the Caesarean, history of vaginal delivery and indication for the prior Caesarean [118].

The model has been successfully validated by this group and in several other cohorts [119–121].

3.8 Conjugate models to predict labour dystocia

Kim et al. in their prospective observational study published in 2010 examined clinical and ultrasonographic parameters for predicting the risk of intrapartum Caesarean delivery in nulliparous women [122].

These investigators recruited 453 women and performed clinical and ultrasonographic assessments at 37 weeks' gestation. Fifty-seven (12.6%) of these participants had an intrapartum Caesarean delivery. They analysed the importance of clinical parameters including maternal age, maternal height, maternal weight and Bishop score. Ultrasonographic parameters documented included foetal biparietal diameter, abdominal circumference, estimated foetal weight, amniotic fluid index and cervical length. Univariate analysis was used to confirm normal distribution. This was conducted using the Student's t-test and Mann-Whitney U test amongst others. Multiple logistic regression analysis was utilised to identify which parameters were most associated with primary Caesarean delivery.

The five most significant parameters in predicting the risk of Caesarean delivery in nulliparous women were as follows: Maternal age OR 1.19 (95% confidence interval [CI], 1.09–1.30], $P < 0.0001$; maternal height (cm) OR 0.89 (95% confidence interval [CI], 0.84–0.95), P 0.001; foetal abdominal circumference (cm) OR 1.55 (95% confidence interval [CI], 1.23–1.97), $P < 0.0001$ and estimated foetal weight (g) OR 1.002 (95% confidence interval [CI], 1.001–1.004), $P < 0.000$. A prediction model was developed based on these significant parameters. The model was constructed using stepwise forward logistic regression analysis of the potential predictors identified and the authors concluded that this could be of benefit in assisting decision-making around the most appropriate mode of delivery for women.

This study was designed as a prospective observational study with a sample size of 453 women. However, it should be noted that the authors did not consider examine BMI as a potential predictor. This has been shown by many studies in the literature, some of which have already been mentioned [98, 123] in this literature review as being highly predictive for intrapartum Caesarean delivery. The authors also cautioned that the predictive performance of the model might be overstated as its measures of discrimination are derived from the same analysis that was used to derive the model. They recommended further studies to validate this model in other study populations.

Mazouni et al. also developed and validated a nomogram to predict the risk of Caesarean delivery in macrosomic infants [124]. This was developed using the data collated from 246 women initially and validated in a further study of 206 women in Marseille, France. Interestingly, this study also included multiparous women. The final key predictors, which were incorporated into the nomogram, were: maternal age ($p = 0.01$), maternal height ($p = 0.02$), parity ($p < 0.001$), and previous Caesarean section ($p = 0.009$). This study did not examine any ultrasonographic details and instead it retrospectively examined the maternal data of women who had delivered a baby >4000 g.

Burke et al. published in 2017 a similar conjugate model [125] that represents the predecessor for the subject of this thesis. The genesis study was a prospective observational study, which recruited 2336 low-risk nulliparous women from the island of Ireland from October 2012 to June 2015. These women attended for ultrasound assessment and collection of maternal anthropometric data from 38 + 0 weeks of pregnancy until 40 + 6 weeks of pregnancy and their delivery outcomes were later collated. Genesis found that five parameters were noted to be the most significant predictors of risk of a nulliparous women undergoing intrapartum Caesarean section delivery. These 5 parameters were advancing maternal age OR, 1.21 (95% confidence interval [CI], 1.09–1.34), $P = .0005$; increasing maternal BMI OR, 1.29 (95% CI, 1.17–1.42), $P < 0.0001$; shorter maternal height OR, 1.72 (95% CI, 1.54–1.92), $P < 0.0001$; larger foetal HC OR, 1.27 (95% CI, 1.13–1.42), $P = 0.0001$; and larger foetal AC OR, 1.23 (95% CI, 1.1–1.37) $P = .0004$.

These five predictors were then used to develop a nomogram to individually calculate each nulliparous woman's risk for requiring intrapartum Caesarean delivery.

4. Conclusions

We have highlighted the benefits of risk prediction models in many aspects of healthcare. We know from our own reading that these models have been developed in the field of obstetrics and particularly with the interest of predicting intrapartum caesarean delivery.

However, we are still awaiting a validated successful model, which may be used in clinical practice. We have also not identified any research studies examining the usage of Artificial Intelligence to aid with risk prediction or any randomised trials reviewing the merits of elective Caesarean delivery versus trial of labour in the event of cephalo-pelvic disproportion.

A focus group amongst expectant first-time mothers in our unit confirmed that women would be keen on the introduction of a risk predictive tool, which would be individualised for each woman. They felt that this would aid them in their decision-making and birth planning.

We can see from other areas of medicine that risk predictive tools are a valuable asset for clinicians in their optimum care of patients. To date, we have not found a risk predictive tool, which is in routine clinical use specifically for predicting intrapartum caesarean delivery.

Conflict of interest

The authors declare no conflict of interest.

Author details

Niamh C. Murphy*, Fionnuala M. Breathnach and Naomi Burke
Royal College of Surgeons in Ireland, Dublin, Ireland

*Address all correspondence to: nmurphy@rcsi.ie

References

[1] Allen VM, O'Connell CM, Baskett TF. Maternal and perinatal morbidity of caesarean delivery at full cervical dilatation compared with caesarean delivery in the first stage of labour. BJOG: An International Journal of Obstetrics and Gynaecology. 2005;**112**(7):986-990

[2] Suja D, Manjusha V, Simi B, Nazeema. Study of maternal outcome of emergency and elective caesarean section in a semi-rural tertiary hospital. National Journal of Medical Research. 2014;**4**(1)

[3] Magann EF, Evans S, Hutchinson M, Collins R, Lanneau G, Morrison JC. Postpartum hemorrhage after cesarean delivery: An analysis of risk factors. Southern Medical Journal. 2005;**98**(7):681-685

[4] Smaill FM, Grivell RM. Antibiotic prophylaxis versus no prophylaxis for preventing infection after cesarean section. The Cochrane Database of Systematic Reviews. 2014;**10**:Cd007482

[5] Loudon JA, Groom KM, Hinkson L, Harrington D, Paterson-Brown S. Changing trends in operative delivery performed at full dilatation over a 10-year period. Journal of Obstetrics and Gynaecology: The Journal of the Institute of Obstetrics and Gynaecology. 2010;**30**(4):370-375

[6] Pergialiotis V, Vlachos DG, Rodolakis A, Haidopoulos D, Thomakos N, Vlachos GD. First versus second stage C/S maternal and neonatal morbidity: A systematic review and meta-analysis. European Journal of Obstetrics, Gynecology, and Reproductive Biology. 2014;**175**:15-24

[7] Yang X-J, Sun S-S. Comparison of maternal and fetal complications in elective and emergency cesarean section: A systematic review and meta-analysis. Archives of Gynecology and Obstetrics. 2017;**296**(3):503-512

[8] Organisation for Economic Co-operation and Development. Caesarean Sections: Health at a Glance 2017: OECD Indicators. OECD Publishing; 2017

[9] The Lancet. Stemming the global caesarean section epidemic. Lancet. 2018;**392**(10155):1279

[10] Martin JA, Hamilton BE, Osterman MJK, Driscoll AK, Drake P. Births: Final data for 2016. National Vital Statistics Reports: From The Centers for Disease Control and Prevention, National Center for Health Statistics, National Vital Statistics System. 2018;**67**(1):1-55

[11] Betran AP, Torloni MR, Zhang J, Ye J, Mikolajczyk R, Deneux-Tharaux C, et al. What is the optimal rate of caesarean section at population level? A systematic review of ecologic studies. Reproductive Health. 2015;**12**:57

[12] Betran AP, Ye J, Moller AB, Zhang J, Gulmezoglu AM, Torloni MR. The increasing trend in caesarean section rates: Global, regional and national estimates: 1990-2014. PLoS One. 2016;**11**(2):e0148343

[13] Ye J, Betran AP, Guerrero Vela M, Souza JP, Zhang J. Searching for the optimal rate of medically necessary cesarean delivery. Birth. 2014;**41**(3):237-244

[14] Betran AP, Temmerman M, Kingdon C, Mohiddin A, Opiyo N, Torloni MR, et al. Interventions to reduce unnecessary caesarean sections in healthy women and babies. Lancet. 2018;**392**(10155):1358-1368

[15] World Health Organization. WHO Statement on Caesarean Section Rates [WHO/RHR/15.02]. Geneva: World Health Organization; 2015

[16] Mazzoni A, Althabe F, Liu NH, Bonotti AM, Gibbons L, Sanchez AJ, et al. Women's preference for caesarean section: A systematic review and meta-analysis of observational studies. BJOG: An International Journal of Obstetrics and Gynaecology. 2011;**118**(4):391-399

[17] Robson SJ, Tan WS, Adeyemi A, Dear KB. Estimating the rate of cesarean section by maternal request: Anonymous survey of obstetricians in Australia. Birth. 2009;**36**(3):208-212

[18] Murray SF. Relation between private health insurance and high rates of caesarean section in Chile: Qualitative and quantitative study. British Medical Journal. 2000;**321**(7275):1501-1505

[19] Safe prevention of the primary cesarean delivery. Obstetric care consensus No. 1. American College of Obstetricians and Gynecologists. Obstetrics and Gynecology. 2014;**123**:693-711

[20] Gamble JA, Creedy DK. Women's preference for a cesarean section: Incidence and associated factors. Birth. 2001;**28**(2):101-110

[21] Hildingsson I, Rådestad I, Rubertsson C, Waldenström U. Few women wish to be delivered by caesarean section. BJOG: An International Journal of Obstetrics and Gynaecology. 2002;**109**(6):618-623

[22] Osis MJ, Padua KS, Duarte GA, Souza TR, Faundes A. The opinion of Brazilian women regarding vaginal labor and cesarean section. International Journal of Gynaecology and Obstetrics: The Official Organ of the International Federation of Gynaecology and Obstetrics. 2001;**75**(Suppl 1):S59-S66

[23] Potter JE, Berquo E, Perpetuo IH, Leal OF, Hopkins K, Souza MR, et al. Unwanted caesarean sections among public and private patients in Brazil: Prospective study. British Medical Journal. 2001;**323**(7322):1155-1158

[24] Angeja AC, Washington AE, Vargas JE, Gomez R, Rojas I, Caughey AB. Chilean women's preferences regarding mode of delivery: Which do they prefer and why? BJOG: An International Journal of Obstetrics and Gynaecology. 2006;**113**(11):1253-1258

[25] Vogenberg FR. Predictive and prognostic models: Implications for healthcare decision-making in a modern recession. American Health & Drug Benefits. 2009;**2**(6):218-222

[26] Perel P, Edwards P, Wentz R, Roberts I. Systematic review of prognostic models in traumatic brain injury. BMC Medical Informatics and Decision Making. 2006;**6**:38

[27] Abu-Hanna A, Lucas PJ. Prognostic models in medicine. AI and statistical approaches. Methods of Information in Medicine. 2001;**40**(1):1-5

[28] Justice AC, Covinsky KE, Berlin JA. Assessing the generalizability of prognostic information. Annals of Internal Medicine. 1999;**130**(6):515-524

[29] Lloyd-Jones DM, Larson MG, Beiser A, Levy D. Lifetime risk of developing coronary heart disease. Lancet. 1999;**353**(9147):89-92

[30] Carlson B. Predictive modeling, sharp lens on near future. Managed Care. 2003;**12**(7):16-21

[31] Kleinrouweler CE, Cheong-See FM, Collins GS, Kwee A, Thangaratinam S, Khan KS, et al. Prognostic models in obstetrics: Available, but far from applicable. American Journal of Obstetrics and Gynecology. 2016;**214**(1):79-90.e36

[32] Apgar V. A proposal for a new method of evaluation of the newborn infant. Current Researches in Anesthesia & Analgesia. 1953;**32**(4):260-267

[33] Bishop EH. Pelvic scoring for elective induction. Obstetrics and Gynecology. 1964;**24**:266-268

[34] Casey BM, McIntire DD, Leveno KJ. The continuing value of the Apgar score for the assessment of newborn infants. The New England Journal of Medicine. 2001;**344**(7):467-471

[35] Finster M, Wood M. The Apgar score has survived the test of time. Anesthesiology. 2005;**102**(4):855-857

[36] James BC. Making it easy to do it right. The New England Journal of Medicine. 2001;**345**(13):991-993

[37] Reilly BM, Evans AT. Translating clinical research into clinical practice: Impact of using prediction rules to make decisions. Annals of Internal Medicine. 2006;**144**(3):201-209

[38] Cheong-See F, Allotey J, Marlin N, Mol BW, Schuit E, Ter Riet G, et al. Prediction models in obstetrics: Understanding the treatment paradox and potential solutions to the threat it poses. BJOG: An International Journal of Obstetrics and Gynaecology. 2016;**123**(7):1060-1064

[39] Rao SC, Chhatriwalla AK, Kennedy KF, Decker CJ, Gialde E, Spertus JA, et al. Pre-procedural estimate of individualized bleeding risk impacts physicians' utilization of bivalirudin during percutaneous coronary intervention. Journal of the American College of Cardiology. 2013;**61**(18):1847-1852

[40] Schuit E, Groenwold RH, Harrell FE Jr, de Kort WL, Kwee A, Mol BW, et al. Unexpected predictor-outcome associations in clinical prediction research: Causes and solutions. Canadian Medical Association Journal. 2013;**185**(10):E499-E505

[41] Thangaratinam S, Allotey J, Marlin N, Dodds J, Cheong-See F, von Dadelszen P, et al. Prediction of complications in early-onset pre-eclampsia [PREP]: Development and external multinational validation of prognostic models. BMC Medicine. 2017;**15**(1):68

[42] Timmerman D, Van Calster B, Testa A, Savelli L, Fischerova D, Froyman W, et al. Predicting the risk of malignancy in adnexal masses based on the simple rules from the international ovarian tumor analysis group. American Journal of Obstetrics and Gynecology. 2016;**214**(4):424-437

[43] Timmerman D, Testa AC, Bourne T, Ameye L, Jurkovic D, Van Holsbeke C, et al. Simple ultrasound-based rules for the diagnosis of ovarian cancer. Ultrasound in Obstetrics & Gynecology. 2008;**31**(6):681-690

[44] Kansagara D, Englander H, Salanitro A, Kagen D, Theobald C, Freeman M, et al. Risk prediction models for hospital readmission: A systematic review. Journal of the American Medical Association. 2011;**306**(15):1688-1698

[45] Jack BW, Chetty VK, Anthony D, Greenwald JL, Sanchez GM, Johnson AE, et al. A reengineered hospital discharge program to decrease rehospitalization: A randomized trial. Annals of Internal Medicine. 2009;**150**(3):178-187

[46] Krumholz HM, Brindis RG, Brush JE, Cohen DJ, Epstein AJ, Furie K, et al. Standards for statistical models used for public reporting of health outcomes: An American Heart Association scientific statement from the quality of care and outcomes research interdisciplinary writing group: Cosponsored by the council on epidemiology and prevention and the stroke council. Endorsed by the American College of Cardiology Foundation. Circulation. 2006;**113**(3):456-462

[47] Toll DB, Janssen KJ, Vergouwe Y, Moons KG. Validation, updating and impact of clinical prediction rules: A review. Journal of Clinical Epidemiology. 2008;**61**(11):1085-1094

[48] Moons KG, Kengne AP, Woodward M, Royston P, Vergouwe Y, Altman DG, et al. Risk prediction models: I. Development, internal validation, and assessing the incremental value of a new [bio]marker. Heart. 2012;**98**(9):683-690

[49] Wilson PW, D'Agostino RB, Levy D, Belanger AM, Silbershatz H, Kannel WB. Prediction of coronary heart disease using risk factor categories. Circulation. 1998;**97**(18):1837-1847

[50] Conroy RM, Pyorala K, Fitzgerald AP, Sans S, Menotti A, De Backer G, et al. Estimation of ten-year risk of fatal cardiovascular disease in Europe: The SCORE project. European Heart Journal. 2003;**24**(11):987-1003

[51] Woodward M, Brindle P, Tunstall-Pedoe H. Adding social deprivation and family history to cardiovascular risk assessment: The ASSIGN score from the Scottish heart health extended cohort [SHHEC]. Heart. 2007;**93**(2):172-176

[52] Nashef SA, Roques F, Michel P, Gauducheau E, Lemeshow S, Salamon R. European system for cardiac operative risk evaluation [EuroSCORE]. European Journal of Cardio-Thoracic Surgery: Official Journal of The European Association for Cardio-Thoracic Surgery. 1999;**16**(1):9-13

[53] Assmann G, Cullen P, Schulte H. Simple scoring scheme for calculating the risk of acute coronary events based on the 10-year follow-up of the prospective cardiovascular Münster [PROCAM] study. Circulation. 2002;**105**(3):310-315

[54] Wells PS, Anderson DR, Bormanis J, Guy F, Mitchell M, Gray L, et al. Value of assessment of pretest probability of deep-vein thrombosis in clinical management. Lancet. 1997;**350**(9094):1795-1798

[55] Lloyd-Jones DM. Cardiovascular risk prediction: Basic concepts, current status, and future directions. Circulation. 2010;**121**(15):1768-1777

[56] Moons KG. Criteria for scientific evaluation of novel markers: A perspective. Clinical Chemistry. 2010;**56**(4):537-541

[57] Steinkamp HJ, Zwicker C, Langer M, Mathe M, Ehritt C, Neumann K, et al. Reactive enlargement of cervical lymph nodes and cervical lymph node metastases: Sonography [M/Q quotient] and computed tomography. Aktuelle Radiologie. 1992;**2**(4):188-195

[58] Cardoso F, Harbeck N, Fallowfield L, Kyriakides S, Senkus E. Locally recurrent or metastatic breast cancer: ESMO clinical practice guidelines for diagnosis, treatment and follow-up. Annals of Oncology: Official Journal of the European Society for Medical Oncology. 2012;**23**(Suppl 7):vii11-vii19

[59] Oostendorp LJ, Stalmeier PF, Donders AR, van der Graaf WT, Ottevanger PB. Efficacy and safety of palliative chemotherapy for patients with advanced breast cancer pretreated with anthracyclines and taxanes: A systematic review. The Lancet Oncology. 2011;**12**(11):1053-1061

[60] Alfarouk KO, Stock CM, Taylor S, Walsh M, Muddathir AK, Verduzco D, et al. Resistance to cancer chemotherapy: Failure in drug response from ADME to P-gp. Cancer Cell International. 2015;**15**:71

[61] Mucaki EJ, Zhao JZL, Lizotte DJ, Rogan PK. Predicting responses to platin chemotherapy agents with biochemically-inspired machine learning. Signal Transduction and Targeted Therapy. 2019;**4**(1):1

[62] Akamatsu N, Nakajima H, Ono M, Miura Y. Increase in acetyl CoA synthetase activity after phenobarbital treatment. Biochemical Pharmacology. 1975;**24**(18):1725-1727

[63] Burrell RA, McGranahan N, Bartek J, Swanton C. The causes and consequences of genetic heterogeneity in cancer evolution. Nature. 2013;**501**(7467):338-345

[64] Block KI, Gyllenhaal C, Lowe L, Amedei A, Amin ARMR, Amin A, et al. Designing a broad-spectrum integrative approach for cancer prevention and treatment. Seminars in Cancer Biology. 2015;**35**(Suppl):S276-s304

[65] Ubels J, Sonneveld P, van Beers EH, Broijl A, van Vliet MH, de Ridder J. Predicting treatment benefit in multiple myeloma through simulation of alternative treatment effects. Nature Communications. 2018;**9**([1]):2943

[66] Howlader N, Noone AM, Krapcho M, Miller D, Brest A, Yu M, et al. SEER Cancer Statistics Review 1975-2015. Bethesda, MD: National Cancer Institute; 2018. Available from: https://seer.cancer.gov/csr/1975_2015/

[67] Lohr JG, Stojanov P, Carter SL, Cruz-Gordillo P, Lawrence MS, Auclair D, et al. Widespread genetic heterogeneity in multiple myeloma: Implications for targeted therapy. Cancer Cell. 2014;**25**(1):91-101

[68] Boyle A, Reddy UM, Landy HJ, Huang C-C, Driggers RW, Laughon SK. Primary cesarean delivery in the United States. Obstetrics and Gynecology. 2013;**122**(1):33-40

[69] Mocanu EV, Greene RA, Byrne BM, Turner MJ. Obstetric and neonatal outcome of babies weighing more than 4.5 kg: An analysis by parity. European Journal of Obstetrics, Gynecology, and Reproductive Biology. 2000;**92**(2):229-233

[70] Shechter Y, Levy A, Wiznitzer A, Zlotnik A, Sheiner E. Obstetric complications in grand and great grand multiparous women. The Journal of Maternal-Fetal & Neonatal Medicine: The Official Journal of The European Association of Perinatal Medicine, The Federation of Asia and Oceania Perinatal Societies, The International Society of Perinatal Obstetricians. 2010;**23**(10):1211-1217

[71] Zhu BP, Grigorescu V, Le T, Lin M, Copeland G, Barone M, et al. Labor dystocia and its association with interpregnancy interval. American Journal of Obstetrics and Gynecology. 2006;**195**(1):121-128

[72] Algovik M, Kivinen K, Peterson H, Westgren M, Kere J. Genetic evidence of multiple loci in dystocia-difficult labour. BMC Medical Genetics. 2010;**11**(1):105

[73] Galvin DM, Burke N, Burke G, Breathnach F, McAuliffe F, Morrison J, et al. 94: Accuracy of prenatal detection of macrosomia >4,000g and outcomes in the absence of intervention: Results of the prospective multicenter genesis study. American Journal of Obstetrics and Gynecology. 2017;**216**(1):S68

[74] Chauhan SP, Grobman WA, Gherman RA, Chauhan VB, Chang G, Magann EF, et al. Suspicion and treatment of the macrosomic fetus: A review. American Journal of Obstetrics and Gynecology. 2005;**193**(2):332-346

[75] Kennelly MM, Anjum R, Lyons S, Burke G. Postpartum fetal head circumference and its influence on labour duration in nullipara. Journal of Obstetrics and Gynaecology: The Journal of The Institute of Obstetrics and Gynaecology. 2003;**23**(5):496-499

[76] Elvander C, Hogberg U, Ekeus C. The influence of fetal head circumference on labor outcome: A population-based register study.

Acta Obstetricia et Gynecologica Scandinavica. 2012;**91**(4):470-475

[77] Valsky DV, Lipschuetz M, Bord A, Eldar I, Messing B, Hochner-Celnikier D, et al. Fetal head circumference and length of second stage of labor are risk factors for levator ani muscle injury, diagnosed by 3-dimensional transperineal ultrasound in primiparous women. American Journal of Obstetrics and Gynecology. 2009;**201**(1):91.e1-91.e7

[78] Caldwell WE, Moloy HC, Anthony D'esopo D. A roentgenologic study of the mechanism of engagement of the fetal head. American Journal of Obstetrics and Gynecology. 1934;**28**(6):824-841

[79] Gardberg M, Laakkonen E, Salevaara M. Intrapartum sonography and persistent occiput posterior position: A study of 408 deliveries. Obstetrics and Gynecology. 1998;**91** (5 Pt 1):746-749

[80] Cunningham FG, Leveno KJ, Bloom SL, Hauth JC, Gilstrap III LC, Wenstrom KD. Williams Obstetrics. 22nd ed. New York: McGraw Hill; 2005

[81] Baskett TF, Calder AA, Arulkumaran S, Munro Kerr's Pr M. Operative Obstetrics. 10th ed. London: Baillie're Tindall; 1982

[82] Akmal S, Kametas N, Tsoi E, Howard R, Nicolaides KH. Ultrasonographic occiput position in early labour in the prediction of caesarean section. BJOG: An International Journal of Obstetrics and Gynaecology. 2004;**111**(6):532-536

[83] Fitzpatrick M, McQuillan K, O'Herlihy C. Influence of persistent occiput posterior position on delivery outcome. Obstetrics and Gynecology. 2001;**98**(6):1027-1031

[84] Ponkey SE, Cohen AP, Heffner LJ, Lieberman E. Persistent fetal occiput posterior position: Obstetric outcomes. Obstetrics and Gynecology. 2003;**101** (5 Pt 1):915-920

[85] Sizer AR, Nirmal DM. Occipitoposterior position: Associated factors and obstetric outcome in nulliparas. Obstetrics and Gynecology. 2000;**96**(5 Pt 1):749-752

[86] Ulset E, Undheim R, Malterud K. Has the obesity epidemic reached Norway? Tidsskrift for den Norske Lægeforening: Tidsskrift for Praktisk Medicin, ny Række. 2007;**127**(1):34-37

[87] Ludford I, Scheil W, Tucker G, Grivell R. Pregnancy outcomes for nulliparous women of advanced maternal age in South Australia, 1998-2008. The Australian and New Zealand Journal of Obstetrics and Gynaecology. 2012;**52**(3):235-241

[88] Timofeev J, Reddy UM, Huang CC, Driggers RW, Landy HJ, Laughon SK. Obstetric complications, neonatal morbidity, and indications for cesarean delivery by maternal age. Obstetrics and Gynecology. 2013;**122**(6):1184-1195

[89] Luke B, Brown MB. Elevated risks of pregnancy complications and adverse outcomes with increasing maternal age. Human Reproduction. 2007;**22**(5):1264-1272

[90] Bayrampour H, Heaman M. Advanced maternal age and the risk of cesarean birth: A systematic review. Birth. 2010;**37**(3):219-226

[91] Bell JS, Campbell DM, Graham WJ, Penney GC, Ryan M, Hall MH. Can obstetric complications explain the high levels of obstetric interventions and maternity service use among older womsen? A retrospective analysis of routinely collected data. BJOG: An International Journal of Obstetrics and Gynaecology. 2001;**108**(9):910-918

[92] Herstad L, Klungsoyr K, Skjaerven R, Tanbo T, Forsen L, Abyholm T, et al. Maternal age and emergency operative deliveries at term: A population-based registry study among low-risk primiparous women. BJOG: An International Journal of Obstetrics and Gynaecology. 2015;**122**(12):1642-1651

[93] Klemetti R, Gissler M, Sainio S, Hemminki E. Associations of maternal age with maternity care use and birth outcomes in primiparous women: A comparison of results in 1991 and 2008 in Finland. BJOG: An International Journal of Obstetrics and Gynaecology. 2014;**121**(3):356-362

[94] Waldenstrom U, Gottvall K, Rasmussen S. Caesarean section in nulliparous women of advanced maternal age has been reduced in Sweden and Norway since the 1970s: A register-based study. BJOG: An International Journal of Obstetrics and Gynaecology. 2012;**119**(13):1591-1596

[95] Herstad L, Klungsoyr K, Skjaerven R, Tanbo T, Eidem I, Forsen L, et al. Maternal age and elective cesarean section in a low-risk population. Acta Obstetricia et Gynecologica Scandinavica. 2012;**91**(7):816-823

[96] Herstad L, Klungsøyr K, Skjærven R, Tanbo T, Forsén L, Åbyholm T, et al. Elective cesarean section or not? Maternal age and risk of adverse outcomes at term: A population-based registry study of low-risk primiparous women. BMC Pregnancy and Childbirth. 2016;**16**:230

[97] Peipert JF, Bracken MB. Maternal age: An independent risk factor for cesarean delivery. Obstetrics and Gynecology. 1993;**81**(2):200-205

[98] Young TK, Woodmansee B. Factors that are associated with cesarean delivery in a large private practice: The importance of prepregnancy body mass index and weight gain. American Journal of Obstetrics and Gynecology. 2002;**187**(2):32-38. Discussion 8-20

[99] Mittal P, Romero R, Tarca AL, Draghici S, Nhan-Chang C-L, Chaiworapongsa T, et al. A molecular signature of an arrest of descent in human parturition. American Journal of Obstetrics and Gynecology. 2011;**204**(2):177.e15-177.e33

[100] Johnson M, Stewart H, Langdon R, Kelly P, Yong L. Women-centred care and caseload models of midwifery. Collegian. 2003;**10**(1):30-34

[101] Homer CS, Davis GK, Brodie PM, Sheehan A, Barclay LM, Wills J, et al. Collaboration in maternity care: A randomised controlled trial comparing community-based continuity of care with standard hospital care. BJOG: An International Journal of Obstetrics and Gynaecology. 2001;**108**(1):16-22

[102] Harvey S, Jarrell J, Brant R, Stainton C, Rach D. A randomized, controlled trial of nurse-midwifery care. Birth. 1996;**23**(3):128-135

[103] Waldenstrom U, Turnbull D. A systematic review comparing continuity of midwifery care with standard maternity services. British Journal of Obstetrics and Gynaecology. 1998;**105**(11):1160-1170

[104] Brocklehurst P, Hardy P, Hollowell J, Linsell L, Macfarlane A, McCourt C, et al. Perinatal and maternal outcomes by planned place of birth for healthy women with low risk pregnancies: The birthplace in England national prospective cohort study. British Medical Journal. 2011;**343**:d7400

[105] AbouZahr CWT, Stanton C, Hill K. Maternal Mortality. World Health Stat Q 199. Vol. 49. 1995. pp. 77-87

[106] Kwast BE. Obstructed labour: Its contribution to maternal mortality. Midwifery. 1992;**8**(1):3-7

[107] Nkata M. Maternal mortality due to obstructed labor. International Journal of Gynecology & Obstetrics. 1997;**57**(1):65-66

[108] Smith JB, Burton NF, Nelson G, Fortney JA, Duale S. Hospital deaths in a high risk obstetric population: Karawa, Zaire. International Journal of Gynaecology and Obstetrics: The Official Organ of the International Federation of Gynaecology and Obstetrics. 1986;**24**(3):225-234

[109] Maharaj D. Assessing cephalopelvic disproportion: Back to the basics. Obstetrical & Gynecological Survey. 2010;**65**(6):387-395

[110] Liselele HB, Boulvain M, Tshibangu KC, Meuris S. Maternal height and external pelvimetry to predict cephalopelvic disproportion in nulliparous African women: A cohort study. BJOG: An International Journal of Obstetrics and Gynaecology. 2000;**107**(8):947-952

[111] Chalmers I, Enkin MKM, editors. Suspected Fetopelvic Disproportion. Oxford: Oxford University Press; 1989

[112] Rozenholc AT, Ako SN, Leke RJ, Boulvain M. The diagnostic accuracy of external pelvimetry and maternal height to predict dystocia in nulliparous women: A study in Cameroon. BJOG: An International Journal of Obstetrics and Gynaecology. 2007;**114**(5):630-635

[113] Morgan MA, Thurnau GR. Efficacy of the fetal-pelvic index in nulliparous women at high risk for fetal-pelvic disproportion. American Journal of Obstetrics and Gynecology. 1992;**166**(3):810-814

[114] Pattinson RC, Cuthbert A, Vannevel V. Pelvimetry for fetal cephalic presentations at or near term for deciding on mode of delivery. The Cochrane Database of Systematic Reviews. 2017;**3**:Cd000161

[115] Abitbol MM, Taylor UB, Castillo I, Rochelson BL. The cephalopelvic disproportion index. Combined fetal sonography and x-ray pelvimetry for early detection of cephalopelvic disproportion. The Journal of Reproductive Medicine. 1991;**36**(5):369-373

[116] Sporri S, Thoeny HC, Raio L, Lachat R, Vock P, Schneider H. MR imaging pelvimetry: A useful adjunct in the treatment of women at risk for dystocia? American Journal of Roentgenology. 2002;**179**(1):137-144

[117] Zaretsky MV, Alexander JM, McIntire DD, Hatab MR, Twickler DM, Leveno KJ. Magnetic resonance imaging pelvimetry and the prediction of labor dystocia. Obstetrics and Gynecology. 2005;**106**(5 Pt 1):919-926

[118] Grobman WA, Lai Y, Landon MB, Spong CY, Leveno KJ, Rouse DJ, et al. Development of a nomogram for prediction of vaginal birth after cesarean delivery. Obstetrics and Gynecology. 2007;**109**(4):806-812

[119] Chaillet N, Bujold E, Dube E, Grobman WA. Validation of a prediction model for vaginal birth after caesarean. Journal of Obstetrics and Gynaecology Canada. 2013;**35**(2):119-124

[120] Costantine MM, Fox K, Byers BD, Mateus J, Ghulmiyyah LM, Blackwell S, et al. Validation of the prediction model for success of vaginal birth after cesarean delivery. Obstetrics and Gynecology. 2009;**114**(5):1029-1033

[121] Maykin MM, Mularz AJ, Lee LK, Valderramos SG. Validation of a prediction model for vaginal birth after Cesarean delivery reveals unexpected success in a diverse American population. AJP Reports. 2017;**7**(1):e31-ee8

[122] Kim SN, Park KH, Jung HJ, Hong JS, Shin DM, Kang WS. Clinical

and sonographic parameters at 37 weeks' gestation for predicting the risk of primary Cesarean delivery in nulliparous women. Ultrasound in Obstetrics & Gynecology. 2010;**36**(4):486-492

[123] Roman H, Goffinet F, Hulsey TF, Newman R, Robillard PY, Hulsey TC. Maternal body mass index at delivery and risk of caesarean due to dystocia in low risk pregnancies. Acta Obstetricia et Gynecologica Scandinavica. 2008;**87**(2):163-170

[124] Mazouni C, Rouzier R, Collette E, Menard JP, Magnin G, Gamerre M, et al. Development and validation of a nomogram to predict the risk of cesarean delivery in macrosomia. Acta Obstetricia et Gynecologica Scandinavica. 2008;**87**(5):518-523

[125] Burke N, Burke G, Breathnach F, McAuliffe F, Morrison JJ, Turner M, et al. Prediction of cesarean delivery in the term nulliparous woman: Results from the prospective, multicenter genesis study. American Journal of Obstetrics and Gynecology. 2017;**216**(6):598.e1-598.e11

Chapter 2

Hemostasis for Massive Hemorrhage during Cesarean Section

Jun Takeda, Shintaro Makino and Satoru Takeda

Abstract

Arterial ligation for massive hemorrhage during cesarean section may often fail to achieve hemostasis because of abundant collateral circulation. In recent years, various methods of hemostasis have been used, of which the most common are compression sutures, uterine balloon tamponade. In cases of massive hemorrhage, patients must be kept in good systemic condition, and local hemostasis must be achieved while paying attention to the possible occurrence of coagulopathy under monitoring of fibrinogen levels. When concomitant coagulopathy is present, local hemostasis is difficult to achieve because of hemorrhagic tendency. In such a case, obstetrical damage control procedures should be performed. First, the hemorrhagic area should be compressed with a towel or balloon, and at the same time, the artery should be blocked or compressed to reduce the blood flow into the uterus. The following resuscitation must also be implemented for warming intervention; blood transfusion to maintain the circulating blood volume; and the treatment of coagulopathy by "triple C supplement," such as combined administration of fresh-frozen plasma and concentrated coagulation factors promptly to obtain a blood fibrinogen level of at least 150–200 mg/dL. If coagulopathy is eliminated, the conventional hemostatic procedures become effective. Hysterectomy is the last measure for hemostasis.

Keywords: cesarean section, compression suture, interventional radiology, massive hemorrhage, obstetrical damage control, uterine balloon tamponade

1. Introduction

The maternal mortality rate in Japan had been decreasing steadily until 2007 (3.1 per 100,000 total births), but thereafter, it showed a fluctuating pattern. The rate was 2.7 per 100,000 total births in 2014 but increased to 3.4 per 100,000 total births in 2016. The major causes of maternal deaths include, in descending order of frequency, critical obstetrical hemorrhage, intracranial hemorrhage, amniotic fluid embolism, aortic vessel disease, respiratory disease, and infectious diseases [1]. Japan has approximately 1 million deliveries per year. A survey conducted by a study group of the Ministry of Health, Labour and Welfare estimated that 4000–5000 cases of pregnancy-related critical illness, if not death, occur every year [2]. Among these cases of critical illness, massive hemorrhage is the most frequent cause and is treated by various hemostatic procedures, hysterectomy, or transcatheter arterial embolization (TAE). An analysis of the patients who survived showed that massive hemorrhage during cesarean section accounted for approximately 70% of all cases [2]. Most cases had placenta previa accreta, bleeding from the surface of the placental separation, or concomitant coagulopathy with hemorrhagic tendency [2, 3]. Therefore, the technique of controlling hemorrhage during cesarean section must be mastered. On the other hand, the widespread use of TAE has made it possible to save the patient's life in most cases of massive hemorrhage after vaginal delivery, unless uterine rupture or some other serious conditions occur [3, 4].

Obstetrical hemorrhage occurs abruptly and in a large quantity. If the amount of bleeding exceeds 2000 ml, disseminated intravascular coagulation (DIC) is likely to occur concomitantly. When coagulopathy is present, adequate uterine contraction may not occur, resulting in atonic hemorrhage, which causes further hemorrhage that leads to a vicious circle of adverse events. In view of this particularity of obstetrical hemorrhage, the Japanese Clinical Practice Guide for Critical Obstetrical Hemorrhage was developed in 2010. The current revised edition of this guideline [5] recommends a new concept of obstetrical transfusion therapy, treatment of coagulopathy, and hemostatic techniques such as compression sutures, intrauterine balloon tamponade, administration of uterotonics and tranexamic acid [3, 5–9]. If coagulopathy is present, the fibrinogen level becomes extremely low, and reversal of hemorrhagic tendency can be achieved only by administration of cryoprecipitate or fibrinogen concentrate or transfusion of fresh-frozen plasma (FFP) [3, 5, 10]. In addition, simulation training for obstetrical emergency care has been conducted widely to promote good team medical care in emergency settings [1].

This chapter provides an outline of hemostatic procedures that should be performed for massive hemorrhage during cesarean section, without hastily adopting hysterectomy. In addition, the methods of transfusion to achieve early hemostasis in order to meet the pathological condition of coagulopathy with hemorrhagic tendency and the procedures for obstetrical damage control in cases with DIC will also be described.

2. Hemostatic strategy for massive hemorrhage during cesarean section

2.1 Systemic management and treatment of hypofibrinogenemia

Once hemorrhage has occurred, it is important not only to determine red blood cell (RBC) count, hemoglobin level, hematocrit value, and biochemical parameters but also to measure plasma fibrinogen levels over time by using a simple rapid fibrinogen measuring instrument as point-of-care testing in order to perform early diagnosis and treatment of coagulopathy [5, 10]. In cases of massive hemorrhage, it may be difficult to assess the accurate amount of bleeding. In many cases, the amount of bleeding is underestimated, and the timing of transfusion may be delayed. Therefore, maintaining the blood pressure such as infusion of large volumes of artificial colloid solution and albumin solution, and quick implementation of temporizing hemostatic procedures such as packing, manual uterine compression, and aortic compression, are important until the access to blood transfusion [3].

If circulatory failure persists despite these procedures or if coagulopathy occurs, transfusion of RBC concentrate alone cannot maintain the sufficient circulation blood volume, on the contrary, it may lead to dilution coagulopathy. Administration of FFP is necessary for achieving the elevation and maintenance of blood pressure and colloid osmotic pressure. It should be noted that if the patient experiences shock, RBC transfusion alone cannot increase blood pressure; FFP and RBC should be administered at a ratio of 1:1 in the same manner as in cases of trauma [3, 5, 10]. In cases of consumption coagulopathy, such as in placenta abruption or amniotic fluid embolism, and coagulopathy following massive hemorrhage, the blood fibrinogen level is often <100 mg/dL. Therefore, elimination of the hemorrhagic tendency requires transfusion of 10–15 units of FFP; usually 15 units of FFP are necessary to increase the blood fibrinogen level by 100 mg/dL. To eliminate the hemorrhagic tendency, rapid transfusion of at least 10 units of FFP, rather than RBC, must be performed. Without this treatment, hemorrhage may persist, and the hemorrhagic tendency may continue for days [11]. The mainstay coagulopathy management is elimination of coagulopathy within 6 h. For this purpose, rapid transfusion of FFP should be performed to obtain a blood fibrinogen level of ≥150–200 mg/dL, and a prothrombin time of ≥70% should be targeted [3, 5, 10, 11]. After these treatments, the FFP/RBC ratio of the total transfusion volume may exceed 2.0 in some cases. If blood of the same type is lacking or there is no time for cross-matching in cases of life-threatening critical hemorrhage, not crossmatched compatible RBC such as type O RBC and type AB FFP should be used without hesitation [5]. Rapid transfusion of FFP may cause asymptomatic (saturation of percutaneous oxygen [SpO_2] of ≤95%) or symptomatic pulmonary edema [5]. Therefore, early treatment with a diuretic, carperitide, or a β-agonist should be provided while monitoring the central venous pressure or SpO_2, or more concentrated blood product, such as fibrinogen concentrate and cryoprecipitate, should be given.

In patients with hypofibrinogenemia, the blood fibrinogen level could be more promptly, more efficiently elevated by administration of 3 g of fibrinogen concentrates (3 g of fibrinogen concentrate is almost equivalent to fibrinogen in 12 units of FFP) or three bags of cryoprecipitate (one bag of cryoprecipitate is derived from approximately 480 ml of FFP) [10–13]. If the patient develops coagulopathy, any other coagulation factors than fibrinogen will also decrease. Therefore, FFP and cryoprecipitate are necessary to maintain the sufficient circulation blood volume and supplement other coagulation factors. As the supplies of fibrinogen concentrate and cryoprecipitate have limitations according to the country and region, "Combined administration of FFP and concentrated coagulation factors (triple C) supplement" has been recommended for treating coagulopathy through efficient administration of these three agents to supplement sufficient coagulation factors, especially fibrinogen, to replace blood volume and to maintain blood pressure and colloid osmotic pressure. Management of massive hemorrhage with a focus on "triple C supplement" never caused hemostatic failure that required hysterectomy in >300 patients with cesarean section in whom placenta abruption was accompanied by coagulopathy.

2.2 Local hemostasis

2.2.1 Hemostasis for the surface of the placental separation

For severe hemorrhage from the surface of the placental separation in cases of placenta previa or placenta accreta, pressure hemostasis with gauze and suture hemostasis have been performed commonly, but these procedures are often unsuccessful in the presence of bleeding from a large area. Although separation of the bladder may be necessary on the anterior wall, the use of a simple suture or Z-suture, piercing the whole myometrium at several sites [3]; a large U-shaped suture; an interrupted circular suture consisting of repeated simple sutures in the entire circumference of the anterior and posterior walls [14]; and a suture of the muscular layer to block blood flow in four directions has been reported [3, 14, 15]. On the other hand, Bakri [16] reported that uterine balloon tamponade was effective for controlling hemorrhage from the surface of separation of the placenta previa. This method is also effective for hemostasis during cesarean section (**Figure 1**) [6].

On the other hand, the success rate of internal iliac artery ligation and uterine artery ligation for uterine bleeding is limited and unsatisfactory, because of marked blood inflows via abundant anastomosis of the peripheral uterine artery from the

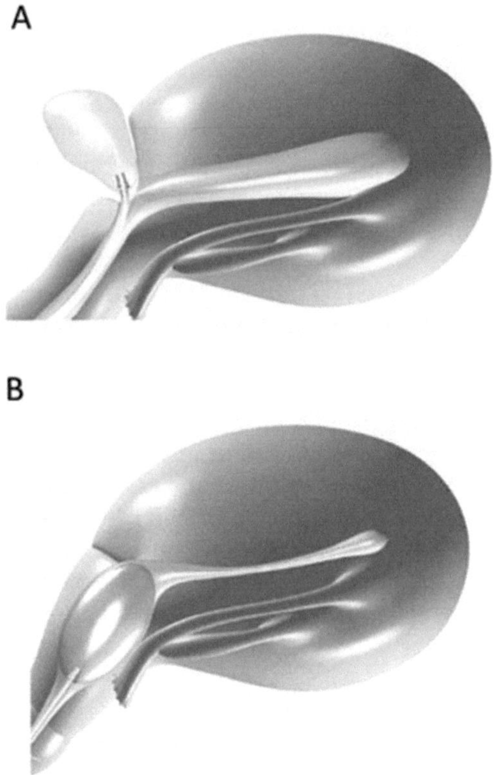

Figure 1.
Balloon insertion during cesarean section. (Produced with permission from Makino et al. [6].) (A) Balloon was inserted through the uterine wound. (B) Eighty to two hundred milliliter of saline is sufficient to achieve hemostasis.

external iliac artery and the aorta [3]. Uterine devascularization, by which the distal portion of uterine artery and the ovarian artery are ligated on the uterine side, has a strong hemostatic effect [17]. However, functional disorders of the uterus and ovaries were reported, such as ovarian dysfunction, oligomenorrhea, endometrial hypoplasia, infertility, uterine cavity adhesions and uterine necrosis [3, 18].

2.2.2 Compression sutures

In cases of atonic hemorrhage, the technique of compression sutures (B-Lynch technique), which was first reported by B-Lynch et al. [19], is used when bimanual compression and administration of uterotonics fail to control bleeding. This technique uses compression of the bleeding surface by joining the anterior and posterior walls of the uterus together. The B-Lynch technique is effective for both hemorrhage from the surface of separation of the placenta previa and atonic hemorrhage and is used for controlling hemorrhage in the lower segment (isthmus) and body of the uterus. As the B-Lynch technique consists of complicated procedures, various modifications have been devised and reported [3, 20]. Various hemostatic techniques include those involving the uterine body or the lower uterine segment (isthmus) alone, or both parts of the uterus for atonic hemorrhage [21, 22].

In our technique of uterine isthmus vertical compression sutures, we used two vertical sutures to achieve pressure hemostasis by sewing the anterior and posterior walls at the uterine isthmus together vertically. This technique is effective for controlling not only hemorrhage in the placenta previa but also atonic hemorrhage

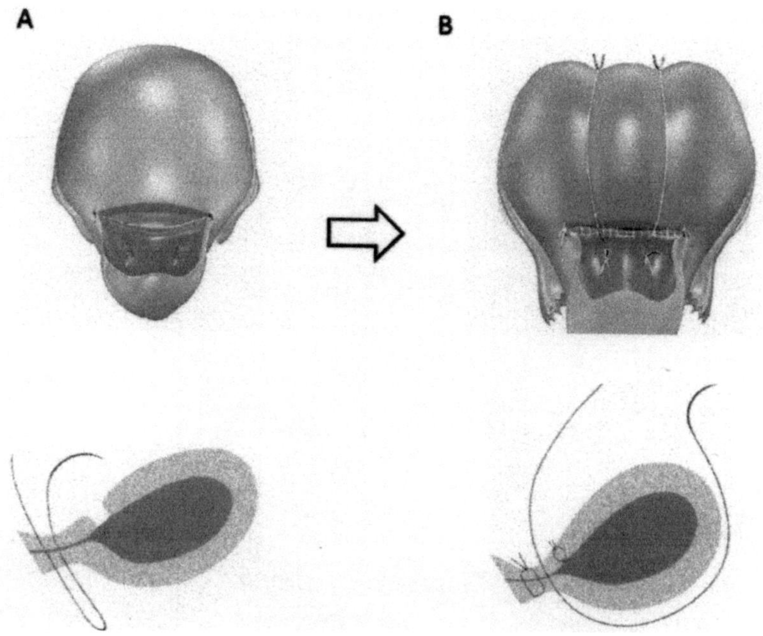

Figure 2.
Double vertical compression sutures. (Produced with permission from Makino et al. [6].) Compression sutures at the uterine isthmus are placed to achieve hemostasis for the atonic bleeding or hemorrhage from a placenta previa. Additional sutures could be placed, as with the modified B-Lynch suture technique, if (A) is not effective.

(**Figure 2**) [3, 6, 21–23]. After exposing the muscular layer in the lower uterus, two stitches piercing the anterior and posterior walls, one each on the right and left sides, were made to place ligation sutures vertically. When the initial vertical compression sutures fail to achieve hemostasis or when there is concomitant coagulopathy, the technique of double vertical compression sutures, a combination of compression sutures and a modified B-Lynch technique, should be used (**Figure 2**) [6, 21]. Synthetic absorbable threads such as Vicryl Rapide® are used. Only two stitches of vertical sutures can also cause pain because of uterine ischemia in some patients, and laparoscopic removal of the thread is required occasionally [24]. This suggests that the procedure of vertical compression sutures not only causes hemostasis by pressing the bleeding surface but also blocks the blood flow entering the uterus from the right and left sides through thread suturing the uterus vertically [22, 25–27]. Therefore, further investigation is necessary as to whether thread removal should be performed even when a quickly absorbable thread is used.

2.2.3 Interventional radiology

Techniques of interventional radiology (IVR) for massive hemorrhage during cesarean section include the arterial balloon occlusion technique by which an arterial balloon catheter is inserted preoperatively to prevent massive hemorrhage and the TAE technique, which is performed intraoperatively in the hybrid operating room [3, 28–30]. The former technique is used in cases of placenta previa accreta and in myomectomy after fetal delivery in cases of pregnancy with a giant myoma. When massive hemorrhage is predicted preoperatively or when hysterectomy is to be performed for placenta accreta, an arterial balloon is placed in the aorta, common iliac artery, and so on. In cases where a procedure that may induce hemorrhage is used or where hemorrhage occurs, the balloon will be inflated to block the arterial

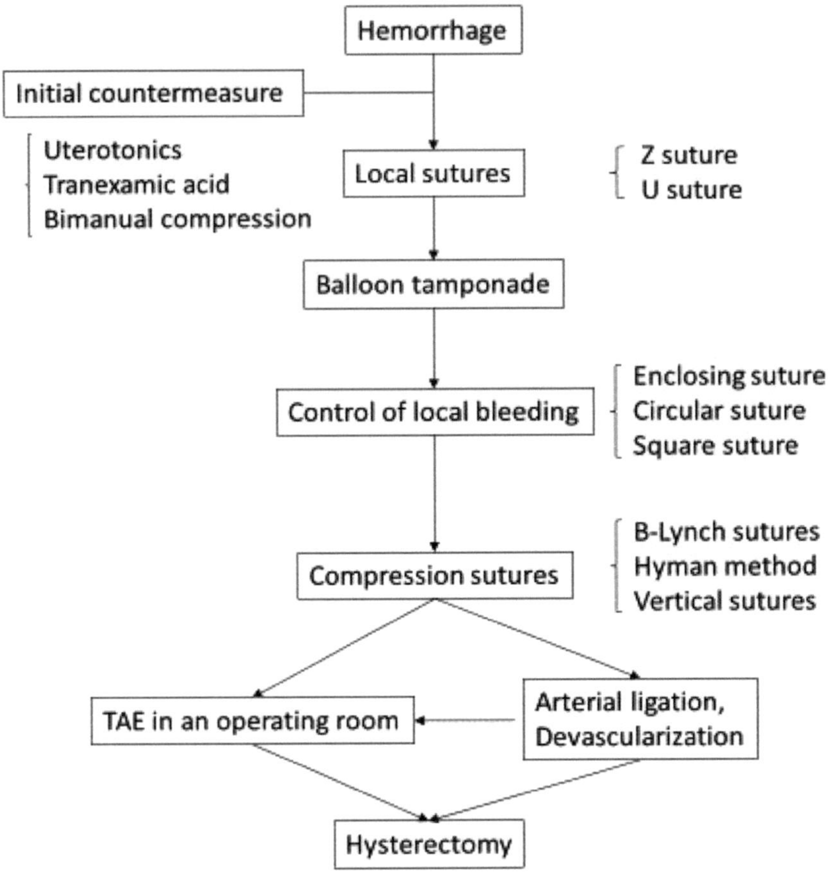

Figure 3.
Hemostatic strategy during cesarean section. (Produced with permission from Takeda et al. [3].) Balloon tamponade or several sutures have priority over TAE or arterial ligation. TAE: transcatheter arterial embolization.

blood flow temporarily to reduce hemorrhage (**Figure 3**) [29–32]. The TAE technique is used for embolization of the bleeding artery in patients operated on in a hybrid operating room equipped with the fluoroscopic apparatus or in surgical patients who are temporarily transferred to a room where a fluoroscopic apparatus is available. This technique is considered useful for patients in whom various local hemostatic procedures have failed to control hemorrhage [28, 29]. However, the association of TAE with prolonged uterine ischemia has become apparent, even when an absorbable embolus such as Spongel® is used [33, 34]. The following complications of TAE have been reported: Asherman syndrome; infertility; ovarian dysfunction (increase in follicle-stimulating hormone levels); endometrial hypoplasia; menstruation disorders (e.g., amenorrhea, menstrual irregularity, oligomenorrhea, and hypomenorrhea); and pregnancy wastage, puerperal massive hemorrhage, placenta accreta, placenta previa, and uterine rupture in subsequent pregnancies [3, 4, 28, 29, 33, 34]. Therefore, TAE and hysterectomy should be recognized as a last measure to be used only when the a forementioned techniques have failed to achieve hemostasis (**Figure 2**) [3].

3. Obstetrical damage control

Hemostasis often cannot be achieved promptly in cases of massive hemorrhage accompanied by coagulopathy. In such cases, damage control surgery (DCS) and resuscitation, which represent the therapeutic concept of life-saving intervention for severe trauma accompanied by massive hemorrhage, should be performed [35, 36]. In the field of emergency medical care, DCS rather than standard surgery is performed in patients having hemorrhagic shock. The primary cause of intraoperative and postoperative deaths in patients with severe trauma accompanied by massive hemorrhage is not loss of blood from the uncontrollable bleeding source but a combination of three abnormalities, namely metabolic acidosis, hypothermia, and blood clotting disorder. These abnormalities are called the lethal triad of death from trauma, resulting from collapse of physiological homeostasis [35, 36]. To treat this condition, gauze or towel packing of the abdomen or the whole pelvis should be performed to provide pressure hemostasis as a part of the DCS [37, 38]. In the meantime, the patient's vital signs and body temperature must be monitored and assessed over time. The patient should be managed to keep in appropriate body temperature. Blood transfusion should be performed to resuscitate the patient from shock and coagulopathy. If hemostasis is judged to be unachievable, the patient should be transported to a higher-level medical facility after performing temporary abdominal closure with intra-abdominal packing [3]. Charoenkwan reported the use of Barki balloon, a method similar to towel packing, to control hemorrhage from the pelvic floor after hysterectomy and from the posterior aspect of the uterus after cesarean section [39, 40].

Hemorrhage may become uncontrollable owing to coagulopathy during cesarean section for cases such as placenta abruption. In these cases, the first measure to be taken is not immediate initiation of hysterectomy. Instead, both application of pressure with a towel or a balloon, and treatment of coagulopathy, in an attempt to prevent the lethal triad of death, may allow avoidance of hysterectomy [11]. Treatment of coagulopathy is accomplished with "triple C supplement" that is a combined administration of FFP and concentrated coagulation factors, such as fibrinogen concentrate, cryoprecipitate, antithrombin, and so on. As the patient's condition may worsen during hysterectomy, pressure should be applied with gauze or a towel after removal of the uterus, and the focus should be on volume replacement, warming of the patient, and treatment of coagulopathy. When the hemorrhagic tendency is improved, drain insertion and abdominal closure are performed. Thus, implementation of resuscitation while the surgical procedure is suspended allows avoidance of unnecessary hysterectomy and hemorrhagic death [3, 11].

In any event, it is important to be familiar with the practice guidelines and emergency care measures for obstetrical critical hemorrhage and to run a simulation of the preparation and actions to be taken in emergency settings. Such simulation training should involve the whole hospital, including not only the obstetrical team consisting of medical and paramedical staff members but also the clerical personnel in charge of the arrangement of blood transfusion, human resources, transfer of patients, and so on. This study emphasizes the importance for obstetrical staff to actively participate in educational programs about maternal emergency in order to prepare for any emergency [1].

4. Conclusion

In cases of massive hemorrhage during cesarean section and in other situations, performing local hemostatic measures while keeping the patient in good systemic condition, monitoring the fibrinogen level, and paying attention to possible occurrence of coagulopathy are important. Minimally invasive hemostasis that has little influence on subsequent pregnancies and deliveries should be attempted [3]. If DIC is present, hemorrhage becomes difficult to control with the usual hemostatic procedures; therefore, "triple C supplement," such as combined administration of concentrated coagulation factors and FFP is necessary in parallel with hemostasis.

If massive hemorrhage occurs during surgery and coagulopathy occurs concomitantly, effective hemostasis cannot be achieved because of the hemorrhagic tendency. In this case, obstetrical damage control should be performed [3, 11]. First, pressure should be applied to the hemorrhagic area with a towel or balloon, and at the same time, arterial blockage or compression should be performed to decrease the blood flow into the uterus. Second, warming of the patient should be implemented. Third, blood transfusion should be performed to maintain the sufficient circulation blood volume. Rapid "triple C supplement" is also important to obtain a blood fibrinogen level of at least 150–200 mg/dL for the treatment of coagulopathy. If coagulopathy is eliminated, the usual balloon tamponade, compression sutures, arterial ligation, and so on become effective. Hysterectomy should be considered as a last hemostatic measure.

Conflict of interest

None.

Author details

Jun Takeda*, Shintaro Makino and Satoru Takeda
Department of Obstetrics and Gynecology, Faculty of Medicine, Juntendo University, Tokyo, Japan

*Address all correspondence to: jtakeda@juntendo.ac.jp

References

[1] Takeda S. Education and training approaches for reducing maternal deaths in Japan. Hypertension Research in Pregnancy. 2018;**6**:15-19. DOI: 10.14390/jsshp.HRP2018-007

[2] Nakabayashi M, Asakura H, Kubo T. Perinatology committee report. Acta Obstetrics and Gynaecology in Japanise. 2007;**59**:1222-1224 in Japanese

[3] Takeda S, Takeda J, Makino S. A minimally invasive hemostatic strategy in obstetrics aiming to preserve uterine function and enhance the safety of subsequent pregnancies. Hypertension Research in Pregnancy. 2019;7. In press. DOI: 10.14390/jsshp.HRP2018-013

[4] Inoue S, Masuyama H, Hiramatsu Y. Multi-Institutional Study Group of Transarterial Embolization for Massive Obstetric Haemorrhage in Chugoku & Shikoku Area Society of obstetrics and Gynecology: Efficacy of transarterial embolisation in the management of post-partum haemorrhage and its impact on subsequent pregnancies. The Australian & New Zealand Journal of Obstetrics & Gynaecology. 2014;**54**(6):541-545. DOI: 10.1111/ajo.12228

[5] Takeda S, Makino S, Takeda J, Kanayama N, Kubo T, Nakai A, et al. Japanese clinical practice guide for critical obstetrical hemorrhage (2017 revision). The Journal of Obstetrics and Gynaecology Research. 2017;**43**(10): 1517-1521. DOI: 10.1111/jog.13417

[6] Makino S, Hirai C, Takeda J, Yorifuji T, Itakura A, Takeda S. Hemostatic technique during cesarean section. Hypertension Research in Pregnancy. 2016;**4**:6-10. DOI: 10.14390/jsshp.HRP2015-008

[7] WOMEN Trial Collaborators. Effect of early tranexamic acid administration on mortality, hysterectomy, and other morbidities in women with post-partum haemorrhage (WOMAN): An international, randomised, double-blind, placebo-controlled trial. Lancet. 2017;**389**:2105-2116. DOI: 10.1016/S0140-6736(17)30638-4

[8] Gayet-Ageron A, Prieto-Merino D, Ker K, et al. Effect of treatment delay on the effectiveness and safety of antifibrinolytics in acute severe haemorrhage: A meta-analysis of individual patient-level data from 40 138 bleeding patients. Lancet. 2018;**391**:125-132. DOI: 10.1016/S0140-6736(17)32455-8

[9] Ahmadzia HK, Phillips JM, Katler QS, James AH. Tranexamic acid for prevention and treatment of postpartum hemorrhage: An update on management and clinical outcomes. Obstetrical & Gynecological Survey. 2018;**73**:587-594. DOI: 10.1097/OGX.0000000000000597

[10] Matsunaga S, Takai Y, Seki H. Fibrinogen for the management of critical obstetric hemorrhage. The Journal of Obstetrics and Gynaecology Research. 2018;**45**:13-21. DOI: 10.1111/jog.13788

[11] Takeda J, Takeda S. Management of disseminated intravascular coagulation associated with placental abruption and measures to improve outcomes. Obstetrics & Gynecology Science. 2019; In press. DOI: 10.5468/ogs.2019

[12] Makino S, Takeda S, Kobayashi T, Murakami M, Kubo T, Hata T, et al. National survey of fibrinogen concentrate usage for post-partum hemorrhage in Japan: Investigated by the Perinatology Committee, Japan Society of Obstetrics and Gynecology. The Journal of Obstetrics and Gynaecology Research. 2015;**41**(8):1155-1160. DOI: 10.1111/jog.12708

[13] Matsunaga S, Takai Y, Nakamura E, Era S, Ono Y, Yamamoto K, et al.

The clinical efficacy of fibrinogen concentrate in massive obstetric haemorrhage with hypofibrinogenaemia. Scientific Reports. 2017;7:46749. DOI: 10.1038/srep46749

[14] Cho JY, Kim SJ, Cha KY, Kay CW, Kim MI, Cha KS. Interrupted circular suture: Bleeding control during cesarean delivery in placenta previa accrete. Obstetrics and Gynecology. 1991;**78**:876-879

[15] Takeda J, Makino S, Matsumura Y, Itakura A, Takeda S. Enclosing sutures technique for control of local bleeding in a case of placenta increta. The Journal of Obstetrics and Gynaecology Research. 2018;**44**(8):1472-1475. DOI: 10.1111/jog.13670

[16] Bakri YN. Uterine tamponade-drain for hemorrhage secondary to placenta previa-accreta. International Journal of Gynaecology and Obstetrics. 1992;**37**:302-303

[17] AbdRabbo SA. Stepwise uterine devascularization: A novel technique for management of uncontrolled post-partum hemorrhage with preservation of the uterus. American Journal of Obstetrics and Gynecology. 1994;**171**:694-700

[18] Roman H, Sentilhes L, Cingotti M, Verspyck E, Marpeau L. Uterine devascularization and subsequent major intrauterine synechiae and ovarian failure. Fertility and Sterility. 2005;**83**:755-757. DOI: 10.1016/j.fertnstert.2004.07.975

[19] B-Lynch C, Coker A, Lawal AH, et al. The B-Lynch surgical technique for the control of massive postpartum haemorrhage: An alternative to hysterectomy? Five cases reported. British Journal of Obstetrics and Gynaecology. 1997;**104**:372-375

[20] Matsubara S, Yano H, Ohkuchi A, Kuwata T, Usui R, Suzuki M. Uterine compression sutures for postpartum hemorrhage: An overview. Acta Obstetricia et Gynecologica Scandinavica. 2013;**92**:378-385. DOI: 10.1111/aogs.12077

[21] Makino S, Tanaka T, Yorifuji T, Koshiishi T, Sugimura M, Takeda S. Double vertical compression sutures: A novel conservative approach to managing post-partum haemorrhage due to placental praevia and atonic bleeding. Australian and New Zealand Journal of Obstetrics and Gynaecology. 2012;**52**:290-292. DOI: 10.1111/j.1479-828X.2012.01422.x

[22] Takeda J, Hiranuma K, Hirayama T, Makino S, Itakura A, Takeda S. The use of medial, wider vertical compression sutures to reduce uterine blood flow for effaced uterine isthmus: A case report. Journal of Obstetrics and Gynaecology. 2018;**38**(6):871-873. DOI: 10.1080/01443615.2017.1387522

[23] Tanaka T, Makino S, Yorifuji T, Saito T, Koshiishi T, Tanaka S, et al. Vertical compression sutures for control of postpartum hemorrhage from a placenta previa in cesarean section—To evaluate the usefulness of this technique. Hypertension Research in Pregnancy. 2014;**2**:21-25. DOI: 10.14390/jsshp.2.21

[24] Takeda J, Kumakiri J, Makino S, Itakura A, Takeda S. Laparoscopic removal of uterine vertical compression sutures. Gynecology and Minimally Invasive Therapy. 2017;**6**(2):73-75. DOI: 10.1016/j.gmit.2016.03.002

[25] Takeda J, Tanaka K, Ohashi R. Uterine isthmus vertical compression suture for controlling uterine corpus bleeding: A possible mechanism of decreasing uterine blood flow. Hypertension Research in Pregnancy. 2016;**4**:45. DOI: 10.14390/jsshp.HRP2015-018

[26] Anorin-Costa C, Mota R, Rebelo C, Silva PT. Uterine compression sutures

for postpartum hemorrhage: Is routine postoperative cavity evaluation needed? Acta Obstetricia et Gynecologica Scandinavica. 2011;**90**:701-706

[27] Liu S, Mathur M, Tagore S. Complications and pregnancy outcome following uterine compression suture for postpartum haemorrhage: A single Centre experience. Journal of Obstetrics and Gynaecology. 2014;**34**(5):383-386. DOI: 10.3109/01443615.2014.895309

[28] Sone M, Nakajima Y, Woodhams R, Shioyama Y, Tsurusaki M, Hiraki T, et al. Interventional radiology for critical hemorrhage in obstetrics: Japanese Society of Interventional Radiology (JSIR) procedural guidelines. Japanese Journal of Radiology. 2015;**33**:233-240. DOI: 10.1007/s11604-015-0399-0

[29] Kyogoku S. Application and methods of arterial embolization for prophylaxis and treatment of massive hemorrhage in obstetric field. In: Takeda S, Kuwatsuru R, editors. Gynecologic and Obstetric Prophylactic Hemostasis by Intra-Arterial Balloon Occlusion. 1st ed. Singapore: Springer; 2018. pp. 9-21. DOI: 10.1007/978-981-10-8833-9

[30] Takeda J, Makino S. Temporary arterial balloon occlusion for obstetrical field. In: Takeda S, Kuwatsuru R, editors. Gynecologic and Obstetric Prophylactic Hemostasis by Intra-Arterial Balloon Occlusion. 1st ed. Singapore: Springer; 2018. pp. 33-39. DOI: 10.1007/978-981-10-8833-9

[31] Shrivastava VK, Nageotte MP. The utilization of interventional radiologic procedures in the surgical management of placenta accrete syndrome. Clinical Obstetrics and Gynecology. 2018;**61**:795-807. DOI: 10.1097/GRF.0000000000000401

[32] Ono Y, Murayama Y, Era S, Matsunaga S, Nagai T, Osada H, et al. Study of the utility and problems of common iliac artery balloon occlusion for placenta previa with accrete. The Journal of Obstetrics and Gynaecology Research. 2018;**44**:456-462. DOI: 10.1111/jog.13550

[33] Takeda J, Makino S, Ota A, Tawada T, Mitsuhashi N, Takeda S. Spontaneous uterine rupture at 32 weeks of gestation after previous uterine artery embolization. The Journal of Obstetrics and Gynaecology Research. 2014;**40**(1):243-246. DOI: 10.1111/jog.12122

[34] Sano Y, Takeda J, Kuroda K, Makino S, Itakura A, Takeda S. Embrittlement of uterus after uterine artery embolization: A case of uterine perforation. Hypertension Research in Pregnancy. 2016;**4**:42-44. DOI: 10.14390/jsshp.HRP2015-017

[35] Moore EE, Burch JM, Franciose RJ, Offner PJ, Biffl WL. Staged physiologic restoration and damage control surgery. World Journal of Surgery. 1998;**22**:1184-1190

[36] Shapiro MB, Jenkins DH, Schwab CW, Rotondo MF. Damage control: Collective review. The Journal of Trauma. 2000;**49**:969-978

[37] Pacheco LD, Lozada MJ, Saade GR, Hankins GDV. Damage-control surgery for obstetric hemorrhage. Obstetrics and Gynecology. 2018;**132**(2):423-427. DOI: 10.1097/AOG.0000000000002743

[38] Yoong W, Lavina A, Ali A, Sivashanmugarajan V, Govind A, McMonagle M. Abdomino-pelvic packing revisited: An often forgotten technique for managing intractable venous obstetric haemorrhage. The Australian & New Zealand Journal of Obstetrics & Gynaecology. 2018;**59**:201-207. DOI: 10.1111/ajo.12909

[39] Charoenkwan K. Use of the Bakri postpartum balloon in a patient with intractable pelvic floor hemorrhage: when other methods failed to stop

postcesarean bleeding, physicians tried something new. American Journal of Obstetrics and Gynecology. 2013;**209**(3):277.e1-277.e5. DOI: 10.1016/j.ajog.2013.06.043

[40] Charoenkwan K. Effective use of the Bakri postpartum balloon for posthysterectomy pelvic floor hemorrhage. American Journal of Obstetrics and Gynecology. 2014;**210**(6):586.e1-586.e3. DOI: 10.1016/j.ajog.2014.03.068

Chapter 3

Maternal and Fetal Risks in Higher Multiple Cesarean Deliveries

Constantin Zwergel and Constantin S. von Kaisenberg

Abstract

The professionalization of women has shifted family planning to increased maternal ages. This has increased the use of assisted reproduction. Therefore, the tolerance toward suboptimal outcome of pregnancy decreases, and self-determined decision-making is on the rise. Once women have made the decision for elective cesarean section in their first pregnancy, subsequent pregnancies may result in multiple cesarean deliveries. This chapter analyzes the risks associated with higher multiple cesarean deliveries, such as bleeding and transfusion, adhesions, bowel and urinary tract injury, and uterus rupture. It also discussed the risks for vaginal birth following cesarean (VBAC) following multiple cesareans. Also there are neonatal risks involved, and women may require specific obstetric anesthesia. The chapter will analyze the risks for the offspring and the mother depending on the number of previous cesarean sections. This may enable detailed counseling of parents before a higher multiple repeat cesarean section is performed.

Keywords: multiple repeat cesarean section, maternal risks, fetal complications, morbidity, outcome

1. Introduction

Cesarean section is a surgical technique of delivery that frequently saves the life of both the mother and the baby. Although many women especially in the Western world have only one or two children, there are many countries and communities in which the availability of effective contraception is limited and larger families are common. The recent World Health Organization (WHO) data on the frequency of cesarean section show that cesarean section has increased dramatically throughout the world in the past two decades [1]. This rise is independent of the stage of development of a country. In addition, the increase in cesarean section rates shows no signs of slowing down. There are at least two significant reasons for this increase, although the phenomenon has not been yet fully understood: the increasing rate in primary cesarean sections and the rapidly decreasing rate of vaginal birth after cesarean section (VBAC) [2]. An increasing rate of cesarean sections results inevitably in a rise of multiple repeat cesarean deliveries.

It is known that multiple cesarean sections are associated with short- and long-term risks for both the mother and the baby [3–7]. There are several significant maternal complications such as visceral injury, uterine rupture, abnormal placentation, hysterectomy, bleeding and transfusions, severe adhesions, etc., most of which increase with an increasing number of repeated cesarean sections. There are also neonatal risks: babies born via multiple repeat cesarean section are more likely to experience breathing difficulties and to require admission to neonatal intensive care [4, 5, 8, 9].

Although cesarean section is now safer than it has ever been before, there are some knowledge gaps, and there is uncertainty among many obstetricians about the risks involved in multiple cesarean sections, especially when the number exceeds four. Thus, we would like to summarize the results of the most important studies investigating maternal and fetal risks in multiple repeat cesarean sections enabling and facilitating the counseling of parents and the decision-making for delivery.

2. Data collection

We did a systematic literature review of PubMed and the Cochrane Database. Search terms used were multiple cesarean section, repeat cesarean delivery, maternal morbidity, neonatal morbidity, maternal and fetal outcome of multiple cesarean section, bladder injury, uterine scar rupture, placenta increta/percreta, hysterectomy, hemorrhage and transfusion, adhesions after repeat cesarean section, vaginal birth after cesarean section, VBAC after cesarean section, and timing of repeat cesarean delivery.

Prior to beginning the search, we defined inclusion and exclusion criteria. Inclusion criteria were randomized controlled trials, cohort studies, case–control studies, systematic reviews, meta-analysis, and the above search terms. Exclusion criteria were comments, letters to the editor, personal communications, and case reports.

The authors selected the articles first through focused review of the abstracts. Eligible studies underwent full text review. We identified a total of 2190 studies of which 1999 were excluded for not meeting either the inclusion criteria or exclusion criteria or for not answering the research question.

A total of 38 studies and 2 Cochrane systematic reviews ranging from 2005 to 2018 were included in the final analysis. All manuscripts were retrieved in electronic PDF format and analyzed in detail.

The references of the most important studies were again checked for eligibility as part of the search strategy. Data from the randomized controlled retrospective trials and Cochrane systematic reviews were extracted by topic, and data were grouped and reanalyzed.

Thus, the result of this chapter is a review of the safety and risks associated with multiple repeat cesarean section for both the mother and the baby. This can be helpful for the counseling of parents and the decision-making of the mode of delivery.

3. Maternal risks

The results of the most important maternal risks of multiple repeat cesarean sections are summarized (**Table 1**). In total eight studies were eligible and were included in this review. Furthermore, each one of the risks is discussed in detail.

The results of **Table 1** demonstrate that the frequency of bowel and bladder injury is about 0.1% with up to three previous cesarean sections and just under 1% thereafter [3–7]. Uterine rupture is <1% up to two cesarean sections but increases thereafter to about 4%. Blood transfusions are common and required in up to 5%. Intensive care does not increase substantially and is less than 2% (and may also be due to underlying diseases). Hysterectomy and placenta accreta are less than 1% for up to three cesarean sections but 2.5–3% in more than four. Severe adhesions are already common in more than one cesarean section.

Maternal risks of multiple repeat cesarean section				
	First CS	**Second CS**	**Third CS**	**≥4 CS**
Bladder injury	0.09% n = 6/6616 [5, 8, 10, 11]	0.06% n = 10/17,378 [3, 5, 8, 10, 11]	0.23% n = 17/7201 [3, 5, 8, 10, 11]	0.81% n = 20/2461 [3, 5, 8, 10, 11]
Bowel injury	0.13% n = 6/6616 [5, 8, 10, 11]	0.09% n = 10/17,378 [3, 5, 8, 10, 11]	0.18% n = 17/7201 [3, 5, 8, 10, 11]	0.85% n = 20/2461 [3, 5, 8, 10, 11]
Uterus rupture	0.43% n = 126/28,810 [8, 12]	0.61% n = 52/8542 [3, 8, 12]	3.71% n = 29/782 [3, 8]	4.34% n = 41/945 [3, 4, 8, 13]
Blood transfusion	4.05% n = 261/6443 [5, 10, 11]	1.58% n = 273/17,280 [3, 5, 10, 11]	2.23% n = 157/7050 [3, 5, 10, 11]	5.35% n = 142/2652 [3, 5, 10, 11, 13, 14]
ICU admission	1.99% n = 127/6374 [3, 8, 10, 11]	0.59% n = 104/17,388 [3, 8, 10, 11]	0.63% n = 45/7106 [3, 8, 10, 11]	1.95% n = 47/2408 [3, 8, 10, 11]
Cesarean hysterectomy	0.69% n = 44/6374 [3, 8, 10, 11]	0.43% n = 75/17,378 [3, 8, 10, 11]	0.91% n = 65/7106 [3, 8, 10, 11]	2.49% n = 66/2652 [3, 8, 10, 11, 13]
Placenta accreta	0.56% n = 46/6374 [8, 10, 11]	0.36% n = 63/17,438 [3, 8, 10, 11]	0.67% n = 48/7106 [3, 8, 10, 11]	2.57% n = 62/2408 [3, 8, 10, 11]
Placenta previa	6.41% n = 398/6201 [10, 11]	1.35% n = 231/17,170 [3, 10, 11]	1.22% n = 85/6955 [3, 10, 11]	2.87% n = 72/2510 [3, 10, 11, 13]
Severe adhesions	0.83% n = 2/242 [5]	7.27% n = 8/110 [5]	20.00% n = 19/95 [5]	15.15% n = 45/297 [5, 13]

Table 1.
Maternal risks associated with an increasing number of repeated cesarean sections.

3.1 Urological and intestinal injury

The results of **Table 1** demonstrate a slightly increased rate of injury of other intraabdominal organs with increased number of repeat cesarean section. Most of the relevant studies identified a significant difference in both bladder and bowel injuries between lower and higher order elective repeat cesarean section [3–7]. Particularly after more than three prior cesarean sections, the risk of any injury rises substantially [15]. This common finding is probably due to the higher rate of severe adhesions after higher order multiple repeat cesarean section. A frozen situs with multiple severe adhesions needs longer operation time and good surgery skills resulting in higher risks of any injury [16]. Overall a bladder or bowel injury is a quite rare complication in women with multiple repeat cesarean sections.

3.2 Uterine scar rupture

Uterine dehiscence or scar rupture is one of the most feared risks in women with multiple repeat cesarean sections. As expected from the usual clinical experience, the dates of **Table 1** show an increased rate of uterine rupture with rising number of repeat cesarean section, again especially in the group of higher order cesarean section (more than three). Surprisingly in reality, most of the analyzed studies confirm this trend but also report that multiple prior cesarean deliveries were not significantly associated with an increased risk for uterine rupture [3, 16, 17]. Between the different studies, the definition and counting of incomplete or complete uterine dehiscence, small membranic uterine scar, and real uterine rupture are heterogeneous. Also a uterine rupture can sometimes not be clearly detected. In conclusion, uterine rupture is apparently an existing risk but does not seem to be critical and significant for up to two previous cesarean sections.

3.3 Hemorrhage

The topic hemorrhage includes different maternal characteristics such as total hemoglobin decrease, blood loss >1500 ml, any blood transfusion, or massive blood transfusion (more than 4 units). Therefore there is inconsistency on the investigated characteristics depending on the definitions used.

The results of the trials show (**Table 1**) that the quantity of any blood transfusion and also the rate of ICU admission are higher in the first cesarean section on the one side and in the higher order repeat cesarean section (≥4) on the other side than the number of transfusion in the second and third cesarean sections [3, 5, 10, 11, 13, 14]. The increased number of blood transfusions and lengthened intensive care hospitalization following the first cesarean section may be explained by the fact that in this cohort, emergency deliveries and more unexpected situations are included, compared with the cohort of the elective second or third cesarean sections.

Some of the analyzed studies pointed out that there is a significant higher rate of blood loss or any blood transfusion especially in the group of more than three repeat cesarean sections [3, 7, 13, 15, 18]. This may be due to a higher rate of adhesions, visceral injury, and possibly abnormal placentation (see also 3.4.). There are a few trials where no differences in blood transfusions between the cohorts could be found [6, 16].

3.4 Abnormal placental invasion and hysterectomy

Abnormal placental invasion included several characteristics: placenta accreta, increta or percreta, and placenta previa. Placenta accreta is a severe obstetric complication characterized by abnormally deep attachment of the placenta. Placenta increta or percreta describes the more invasive placental attachment to the uterine wall, whereas placenta previa locks the natural birth canal. These placental variations can lead to cesarean hysterectomy and/or a life-threatening maternal hemorrhage.

Like with the other maternal risks, a higher order repeat cesarean section (more than three) means a significant higher rate of placenta praevia, placenta accreta, and hysterectomy (**Table 1**) [3, 8, 10, 11].

Placenta accreta is probably the most clinically significant maternal morbidity subsequent to cesarean delivery because of the association with life-threatening hemorrhage that frequently results in peripartum hysterectomy, cystectomy, and also iatrogenic preterm birth [10, 19–21]. The increase of the incidence of placenta accreta seems to be directly related to the increasing number of multiple cesarean deliveries and is therefore associated with maternal and perinatal morbidities [7, 10, 11].

The incidence of placenta previa also rises together with increased number of cesarean section [3, 8, 10, 11, 22]. Another study pointed out that the rate of placenta previa increased from nearly 1% with one previous cesarean section to about 2.8% with more than three cesarean deliveries [7]. Our results demonstrate (**Table 1**) that even a single prior cesarean delivery can increase the risk for placenta previa [23].

It is also interesting that compared with women with placenta previa and no previous cesarean section, women with placenta previa and more than three cesarean deliveries had a statistically significant increased risk of accreta (3.3–4% vs. 50–67%), hysterectomy (0.7–4% vs. 50–67%), and composite maternal morbidity (15% vs. 83%) [7].

As explained above, placenta previa and placenta accreta were found to be one of the most important risk factors in terms of the need for hysterectomy [19]. Therefore, the rate of hysterectomy after multiple repeat cesarean section rises parallel to the rate of placenta previa and accreta [3, 8, 10, 11, 13].

Altogether the results suggest that abnormal placentation is one of the most significant factors by analyzing the adverse maternal outcome after multiple cesarean section.

3.5 Long-term complications

Long-term complications are essentially due to the risk of severe adhesions after multiple cesarean sections (**Figure 1**). Adhesions can be the consequence of nearly every operation and can represent a serious problem for the delivery of women with multiple repeat cesarean sections.

The results of **Table 1** show that severe adhesions increased parallel to the number of performed repeat cesarean section [10, 24–26]. Especially the rise of the adhesions' rate after more than three cesarean sections is dramatical. Both the incidence and severity of adhesions have been demonstrated to increase with increasing numbers of cesarean deliveries. Adhesions have been also associated with increased operative time, increased blood loss, and increased risk of visceral injury.

Altogether, the rate of severe adhesions after multiple repeat cesarean section is one of the most important keys for maternal outcome after multiple repeat cesarean section.

In summary of the maternal outcome, the risk of some rare but serious maternal morbidities such as visceral injury, hemorrhage, abnormal placentation, hysterectomy, or severe adhesions is importantly increased with the number of multiple repeat cesarean section. There is no clear absolute threshold for the number of cesarean sections, but a total of four or more cesarean deliveries was identified as the critical level for most of the major complications.

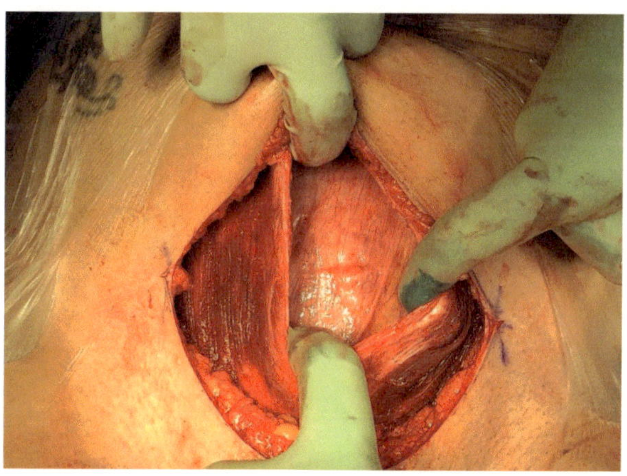

Figure 1.
The Omentum majus is adherent to the anterior uterine wall in a women with three prior cesarean sections (with permission).

4. Fetal risks

Multiple cesarean section may have consequences not only for the maternal but also for the neonatal outcome. Unfortunately, most of the analyzed studies about the risks of multiple cesarean sections place the focus on the mother. Data about the fetal outcome depending on an increased number of cesarean sections are limited. **Table 2** shows an overview for some results of fetal risks in multiple repeat cesarean sections.

There are only 4 studies with a total of 2895 babies that could be looked at [4, 5, 8, 9]. Altogether, there are no significant differences in adverse Apgar score, neonatal intensive care admission, and complications in the neonatal outcome between the groups of lower and higher order repeated cesarean sections. It seems that the neonatal outcome is related to the number of repeat cesarean sections; only some nonsignificant trends were found for adverse fetal outcome. Furthermore, there was no difference in the rate of perinatal death in women with prior cesarean section versus vaginal delivery [27]. More detailed results of neonatal characteristics such as asphyxia, pH-values, fetal defects, and short- and long-term neurological outcome investigating the association with the numbers of repeat cesarean sections could not be found.

There are some studies describing that previous cesarean delivery is associated with an increased risk of preterm birth and small-for-gestational-age fetuses relative to women with no previous cesarean [28, 29]. One trial pointed out that neonates of mothers having multiple repeat cesarean sections were significantly more likely to be born prior to 37 weeks of gestation and therefore had higher rates of complications and admissions, especially adverse respiratory outcome (see also 7) [4]. This aspect may be based on a higher risk potential of women with multiple prior cesarean section (e.g., higher mean maternal age, gravidity, and parity of women who had more than one prior cesarean [5]) and therefore the clinical decision for a preterm elective repeat cesarean section. Preterm birth and fetal growth restriction may also be due to an increased risk of abnormal placentation and uteroplacental dysfunction in association with a prior cesarean section [28].

In conclusion, the results suggest that adverse neonatal outcome depends more on the mode and the timing of delivery than on the number of repeat cesarean section.

Fetal risks of multiple repeat cesarean section				
	First CS	**Second CS**	**Third CS**	**≥4 CS**
Admission to NICU*	13.97% n = 58/415 [5, 8]	20.31% n = 588/2895 [5, 8, 9]	17.70% n = 154/870 [5, 8, 9]	15.81% n = 68/430 [4, 5, 8, 9]
5-min Apgar < 5	9.39% n = 39/415 [5, 8]	2.11% n = 61/2895 [5, 8, 9]	2.18% n = 19/870 [5, 8, 9]	4.49% n = 15/334 [5, 8, 9]
Complications** in fetal outcome	n.k.	21.24% n = 816/3841 [5, 8, 10, 11]	23.07% n = 218/945 [3, 5, 8, 10, 11]	19.56% n = 62/317 [3, 5, 8, 10, 11]

**Neonatal intensive care unit.*
***Intraventricular hemorrhage, severe jaundice, severe infection, hypoxic ischemic encephalopathy.*

Table 2.
Fetal risks associated with an increasing number of repeated cesarean section.

5. Risks in higher order multiple cesarean sections

Cesarean deliveries by women with more than four prior cesarean sections are very rare and are exceptional cases. Usually the third or fourth cesarean section is combined with tubal ligation. However, in some countries or religious groups with large families and by self-determined decision-making, very high order repeat cesarean deliveries can be observed, in particular if contraception is not desired. Therefore it is critical to know how dangerous it is to perform more than four repeat cesarean sections.

There are not many studies describing women undergoing five or higher multiple cesarean sections. One study with 940 cases demonstrated an increase of the risks of all major complications, and dense adhesions were commonly noticed at cesarean delivery, but only eight women had more than four multiple cesarean deliveries [24]. Another study with a total of 318 women investigated especially the risks of higher order (5–9) repeat cesarean sections and identified no difference in maternal and fetal risks between the group of lower (<4) and higher (>4) repeat cesarean section except for an extended operation time and an increased rate of severe adhesions [16].

As shown in Chapter 4 (maternal risks), multiple cesarean deliveries are in general associated with more adhesions and increased blood loss than only one planned cesarean section. It can therefore be concluded that the surgery and management of higher order (>4) repeat cesarean sections are more difficult and require more planning and operation time and skills. One study with a total of 5007 women pointed out that vertical skin incision in these cases is not associated with improved maternal and fetal outcome [9]. Furthermore, the results of another study suggest that the risks of an urgent multiple cesarean section are in the range of elective multiple cesarean section [6, 18]. There were, however, differences for myometrium herniation during this cesarean section, a need for drainage following surgery, and postoperative fever as well as hospitalization (days), which was held due to the urgency.

6. VBAC and the number of repeat cesarean section

Clinical decision-making for women following multiple prior cesarean deliveries is influenced by limited evidence and the expectations of the mother. Vaginal birth after multiple cesarean deliveries can be an option if women are eligible. In order to provide the currently best available evidence, we extracted and regrouped information from four trials (**Table 3**).

A meta-analysis of 20 studies compared the success rate—and the associated adverse maternal and fetal outcomes of vaginal birth—after one and two cesarean sections (VBAC-1/VBAC-2) with a further repeat multiple cesarean section [30]. Women requesting a trial of labor following two cesarean sections should be informed of a success rate for vaginal delivery of 71.7%, a uterine rupture rate of 1.36%, and of a similar maternal morbidity in both groups. Maternal morbidity of VBAC-2 is comparable to that of multiple cesarean sections. The neonatal morbidity data were too limited to draw valid conclusions [30].

Another trial pointed out that women with three or more prior cesareans who attempt VBAC have similar success rates and maternal morbidity as those with only one prior cesarean, as well as those delivered by elective repeat cesarean [31].

There are also two systematic Cochrane reviews showing no statistically significant differences between a planned repeat cesarean birth and a planned vaginal birth after a cesarean section [32, 33].

Delivery	VBAC successes	Uterine rupture	Hysterectomy	Transfusion
VBAC 1	76.50% n = 38,814/50,685 [30]	0.72% n = 372/50,685 [30]	0.19% n = 42/50,685 [30]	1.21% n = 358/50,685 [30]
Second CS	–	0.61% n = 52/8542 [3, 8, 12]	0.43% n = 75/17,378 [3, 8, 10, 11]	1.58% n = 273/17,280 [3, 5, 10, 11]
VBAC 2	71.70% n = 4064/5666 [30]	1.36% n = 74/5421 [30]	0.56% n = 14/2512 [30]	2.01% n = 39/5666 [30]
Third CS	–	3.71% n = 29/782 [3, 8]	0.91% n = 65/7106 [3, 8, 10, 11]	2.23% n = 157/7050 [3, 5, 10, 11]
VBAC > 2	79.77% n = 71/89 [31]	0.00% n = 0/89 [31]	n.k.	2.20% n = 2/89 [31]
≥4 CS	–	4.34% n = 41/945 [3, 4, 8, 13]	2.49% n = 66/2652 [3, 8, 10, 11, 13]	5.35% n = 142/2652 [3, 5, 10, 11, 13, 14]

VBAC1/VBAC2 = vaginal birth after one/two cesarean sections; CS = cesarean section

Table 3.
Maternal outcome of vaginal birth following multiple cesarean section for VBAC versus a setting of increasing higher multiple repeat cesarean sections.

In conclusion, there was no difference in the maternal morbidity of women with multiple prior cesareans for the mode of delivery in these studies. A history of multiple cesarean deliveries is not associated with an increased rate of uterine rupture in women attempting vaginal birth compared with those with a single prior operation (**Table 3**). However, when looking at uterine rupture alone, the risks increase with each cesarean section (>2 CS: 3.71% and >3 CS: 4.34%).

In conclusion, vaginal birth after multiple cesarean deliveries remains an option for eligible women.

7. Timing of elective repeat cesarean section

In clinical practice obstetricians have to decide when best to perform an elective repeat cesarean delivery. For the decision-making, it is interesting to have knowledge on the gestation with the best neonatal and maternal outcomes. We found five studies in total to be analyzed.

Three retrospective studies with a total of 48,757 women were identified comparing the neonatal risks at repeat cesarean delivery before and after 39 weeks of gestation [34–36]. In general elective repeat cesarean sections between 37 and 39 weeks are associated with a higher neonatal morbidity. Especially the rates of adverse respiratory outcomes and mechanical ventilation were increased. Neonates born before 39 weeks of gestation have significant more respiratory distress syndromes. Additionally the risks of newborn sepsis, hypoglycemia, admission to the neonatal ICU, and hospitalization are also higher in the group with a repeat cesarean section before 39 weeks [36].

Another study demonstrated increased costs through increasing adverse neonatal outcomes because of elective repeat cesarean deliveries at 37 or 38 weeks [37].

On the opposite side, the elective cesarean delivery at 39 weeks seems to be associated with better neonatal outcome in comparison to a later timing of delivery [34].

Altogether our findings suggest that from the neonatal point of view, there are benefits to waiting until 39 weeks of gestation to perform an elective repeat cesarean delivery.

To achieve the prolongation of the pregnancy until 39 weeks for the neonatal benefit, it is important to know if an elective repeat cesarean section at this time is also of benefit for the maternal outcome. The results of three studies with a total of 37.938 women show that an elective repeat cesarean delivery at 37 or 38 weeks is not associated with decreased maternal morbidity [34, 35, 38]. In comparison to the group of elective delivery at 39 weeks, there was no significant difference in uterine scar rupture, estimated blood loss, hysterectomy, or other maternal complications.

Additionally one study pointed out that elective cesarean delivery at 37 weeks had significantly higher risks of a prolonged (>5 days) maternal hospitalization [38].

Although a cesarean section before 39 weeks has a similar rate of risks for women with multiple repeated cesarean sections as the delivery after 39 weeks, the elective repeat cesarean section at 37 or 38 weeks exposes the neonate to an unnecessary increased risk of respiratory distress syndromes.

In conclusion, if there are no other medical indications for an earlier delivery, 39 weeks of gestation is apparently the optimal timing for repeat cesarean delivery yielding both the best neonatal and maternal outcome.

8. Summary

- The risks of rare but potentially serious maternal morbidities such as visceral injury, hemorrhage, abnormal placentation, hysterectomy, or severe adhesions importantly increased with the number of multiple repeat cesarean sections.

- Adverse neonatal outcome depends more on the mode and the timing of delivery than on the numbers of repeat cesarean sections.

- There is no clear absolute threshold for a safe number of previous cesarean sections, but a total of four or more cesarean deliveries was identified as the critical level for most of the major complications to be substantially increased.

- Repeat cesarean delivery is done best at 39 weeks yielding the best outcome for both the mother and baby.

- Vaginal birth after multiple cesarean deliveries remains an option for eligible women.

Author details

Constantin Zwergel and Constantin S. von Kaisenberg*
Department of Obstetrics, Gynecology and Reproductive Medicine, Hannover Medical School, Hannover, Germany

*Address all correspondence to: vonkaisenberg.constantin@mh-hannover.de

References

[1] World Health Organization Human Reproduction Programme. WHO statement on caesarean section rates. Reproductive Health Matters. 2015;**23**(45):149-150

[2] MacDorman MF, Menacker F, Declercq E. Cesarean birth in the United States: Epidemiology, trends, and outcomes. Clinics in Perinatology. 2008;**35**(2):293-307

[3] Kaplanoglu M et al. Effect of multiple repeat cesarean sections on maternal morbidity: Data from Southeast Turkey. Medical Science Monitor. 2015;**21**:1447-1453

[4] Cook JR et al. Multiple repeat caesarean section in the UK: Incidence and consequences to mother and child. A national, prospective, cohort study. BJOG. 2013;**120**(1):85-91

[5] Ozcan S et al. Multiple repeat cesarean delivery is associated with increased maternal morbidity irrespective of placenta accreta. European Review for Medical and Pharmacological Sciences. 2015;**19**(11):1959-1963

[6] Zia S, Rafique M. Intra-operative complications increase with successive number of cesarean sections: Myth or fact? Obstetrics & Gynecology Science. 2014;**57**(3):187-192

[7] Marshall NE, Fu R, Guise JM. Impact of multiple cesarean deliveries on maternal morbidity: A systematic review. American Journal of Obstetrics and Gynecology. 2011;**205**(3):262 e1-262 e8

[8] Arlier S et al. Incidence of adhesions and maternal and neonatal morbidity after repeat cesarean section. Archives of Gynecology and Obstetrics. 2017;**295**(2):303-311

[9] Palatnik A, Grobman WA. The association of skin-incision type at cesarean with maternal and neonatal morbidity for women with multiple prior cesarean deliveries. European Journal of Obstetrics, Gynecology, and Reproductive Biology. 2015;**191**:121-124

[10] Clark EA, Silver RM. Long-term maternal morbidity associated with repeat cesarean delivery. American Journal of Obstetrics and Gynecology. 2011;**205**(6 Suppl):S2-S10

[11] Silver RM. Delivery after previous cesarean: Long-term maternal outcomes. Seminars in Perinatology. 2010;**34**(4):258-266

[12] Motomura K et al. Scientific Reports. 2017;**7**:44093

[13] Biler A et al. Is it safe to have multiple repeat cesarean sections? A high volume tertiary care center experience. Pakistan Journal of Medical Sciences. 2017;**33**(5):1074-1079

[14] Cook JR, Knight M, Dhanjal MK. Multiple repeat caesarean section in the UK: Incidence and consequences to mother and child. A national, prospective cohort study—Authors' reply. BJOG. 2013;**120**(9):1155

[15] Abdelazim I, Alanwar A, Svetlana S, Sakiyeva K, Farghali M, Mohamed M, et al. Complications associated with higher order compared to lower order cesarean sections. The Journal of Maternal-Fetal & Neonatal Medicine. 21 Nov. 2018:1-161. DOI: 10.1080/14767058.2018.1551352. [Epub ahead of print]

[16] Rashid M, Rashid RS. Higher order repeat caesarean sections: How safe are five or more? BJOG. 2004;**111**(10):1090-1094

[17] Landon MB et al. Risk of uterine rupture with a trial of labor in women

with multiple and single prior cesarean delivery. Obstetrics and Gynecology. 2006;**108**(1):12-20

[18] Gedikbasi A et al. Multiple repeated cesarean deliveries: Operative complications in the fourth and fifth surgeries in urgent and elective cases. Taiwanese Journal of Obstetrics & Gynecology. 2010;**49**(4):425-431

[19] Shellhaas CS et al. The frequency and complication rates of hysterectomy accompanying cesarean delivery. Obstetrics and Gynecology. 2009;**114** (2 Pt 1):224-229

[20] Eller AG et al. Optimal management strategies for placenta accreta. BJOG. 2009;**116**(5):648-654

[21] Bauer ST, Bonanno C. Abnormal placentation. Seminars in Perinatology. 2009;**33**(2):88-96

[22] Getahun D et al. Previous cesarean delivery and risks of placenta previa and placental abruption. Obstetrics and Gynecology. 2006;**107**(4):771-778

[23] Lydon-Rochelle M et al. First-birth cesarean and placental abruption or previa at second birth(1). Obstetrics and Gynecology. 2001;**97**(5 Pt 1):765-769

[24] Nisenblat V et al. Maternal complications associated with multiple cesarean deliveries. Obstetrics and Gynecology. 2006;**108**(1):21-26

[25] Tulandi T et al. Adhesion development and morbidity after repeat cesarean delivery. American Journal of Obstetrics and Gynecology. 2009;**201**(1):56 e1-56 e6

[26] Morales KJ, Gordon MC, Bates GW Jr. Postcesarean delivery adhesions associated with delayed delivery of infant. American Journal of Obstetrics and Gynecology. 2007;**196**(5):461 e1-461 e6

[27] Hemminki E, Shelley J, Gissler M. Mode of delivery and problems in subsequent births: A register-based study from Finland. American Journal of Obstetrics and Gynecology. 2005;**193**(1):169-177

[28] Smith GC, Pell JP, Dobbie R. Caesarean section and risk of unexplained stillbirth in subsequent pregnancy. Lancet. 2003;**362**(9398):1779-1784

[29] Kennare R et al. Risks of adverse outcomes in the next birth after a first cesarean delivery. Obstetrics and Gynecology. 2007;**109**(2 Pt 1):270-276

[30] Tahseen S, Griffiths M. Vaginal birth after two caesarean sections (VBAC-2)-a systematic review with meta-analysis of success rate and adverse outcomes of VBAC-2 versus VBAC-1 and repeat (third) caesarean sections. BJOG. 2010;**117**(1):5-19

[31] Cahill AG et al. Vaginal birth after caesarean for women with three or more prior caesareans: Assessing safety and success. BJOG. 2010;**117**(4):422-427

[32] Dodd JM et al. Planned elective repeat caesarean section versus planned vaginal birth for women with a previous caesarean birth. Cochrane Database of Systematic Reviews. 2013;**12**:CD004224

[33] Horey D et al. Interventions for supporting pregnant women's decision-making about mode of birth after a caesarean. Cochrane Database of Systematic Reviews. 2013;7:CD010041

[34] Chiossi G et al. Timing of delivery and adverse outcomes in term singleton repeat cesarean deliveries. Obstetrics and Gynecology. 2013;**121**(3):561-569

[35] Hamadneh J et al. Association between timing of elective cesarean delivery and adverse outcomes among women with at least two previous cesareans. International

Journal of Gynaecology and Obstetrics. 2017;**137**(1):51-56

[36] Tita AT et al. Timing of elective repeat cesarean delivery at term and neonatal outcomes. The New England Journal of Medicine. 2009;**360**(2):111-120

[37] Robinson CJ et al. Timing of elective repeat cesarean delivery at term and neonatal outcomes: A cost analysis. American Journal of Obstetrics and Gynecology. 2010;**202**(6):632 e1-632 e6

[38] Tita AT et al. Timing of elective repeat cesarean delivery at term and maternal perioperative outcomes. Obstetrics and Gynecology. 2011;**117**(2 Pt 1):280-286

Chapter 4

Cesarean Scar Defect Manifestations during Pregnancy and Delivery

Ospan Mynbaev, Ioannis Kosmas, Zhongjie Shi, Sergei Firichenko, Avinoam Tzabari, Lin Ma, Leila Kindarova, Tatiana Babenko, Styliani Salta, Antonio Malvasi, Ivano Raimondo, Andrea Tinelli, Victor Gomel and Michael Stark

Abstract

The cesarean scar is a significant risk factor for the following pregnancies and especially deliveries. In this chapter, we discussed the diagnosis, incidence, detection, manifestations, and prognosis of pregnancy and delivery with cesarean scars. A systematic review of current literature showed that a manifestation of cesarean scars during the following pregnancies is not predictable, in general, although modern visualization technologies could reveal some specific features of scar defects that are associated with complications during pregnancy and delivery. However, there is no factor, which could serve as the main prognostic guide for obstetricians to make a decision for VBAC, thus Edwin Cragin's phrase "once a cesarean, always a cesarean" has represented the essential healthcare issue over the century. At the moment, the most reasonable measurements to prevent uterine scar complications are reducing the rate of Cesarean Sections, opening the uterus transversely in the lower segment, and stitching the uterus with one layer only continuously using a big needle preferable by Stark technique of Cesarean section.

Keywords: cesarean scar, pregnancy, delivery

1. Introduction

Cesarean scar defect is diagnosed in the presence of a hypo-echogenic indentation (a filling defect) within the myometrium of the lower uterine segment on the site of a previous cesarean incision that is communicated with the uterine or cervical cavity [1]. The cesarean scar is a significant risk factor for the following pregnancies and especially for future deliveries. All pregnancies in women who experienced previous cesarean sections (CSs) are considered to be at a high-risk due to the possibility of scar defect complications.

2. The manifestation of cesarean scar pregnancy

Au et al. [1] reviewed the data of 183 women with the previous CSs with the aim to determine whether the cesarean scar defect parameters assessed by transvaginal ultrasonography (TVS) might affect the outcome of early termination of pregnancy (TOP) with mifepristone-misoprostol. Once identified, the myometrial defects were evaluated in the longitudinal plane (**Figure 1A**) by recording the following parameters: scar width (length of the widest gap along the isthmico-cervical canal), scar depth (vertical distance between base and apex of the defect), thickness of the residual myometrium over the defect, and thickness of the myometrium adjacent to the defect (**Figure 1B**) [1].

The authors also calculated the ratio of the residual myometrial thickness over the defect and the adjacent myometrial thickness, and the women were divided into three subgroups accordingly (myometrial thickness ratio <30%, 30–70%, and >70%) [1]. The intrauterine gestational age was determined by measuring the crown-rump length at TVS. When it was estimated 10–15 mm, it was decided as a gestational age of 42–56 days [1]. A successful TOP was defined as absence of an intrauterine gestational sac at TVS without surgical intervention, whereas a failed TOP was defined as a need for D&C after a complete medical regimen for any of the following reasons: (a) excessive vaginal bleeding; (b) intractable lower abdominal pain; (c) suspected septic TOP; (d) persistent incomplete TOP; or (e) ongoing pregnancy in follow-up visits [1].

The authors demonstrated that the parity, previous TOP, and the number of previous CSs were not associated with failed TOP, although the proportion of women with cesarean scar defects was significantly higher in the group with TOP failure as compared with the successful TOP group (53.5 vs. 25.7%). However, after adjusting for these three parameters, on multivariate logistic regression analysis, the women with a defective scar had similar odds of failed TOP compared with those who had an intact scar (**Table 1**) [1].

The significant value of this study is the defect size comparison between women with successful and those with failed TOP among 59 women with cesarean scar defects (**Table 2**) [1]. The authors demonstrated that the median defect width was not significantly different between women with successful and those with failed TOP, but the median defect depth was considerably larger in women with failed TOP if compared with those with successful TOP [1]. The median myometrial

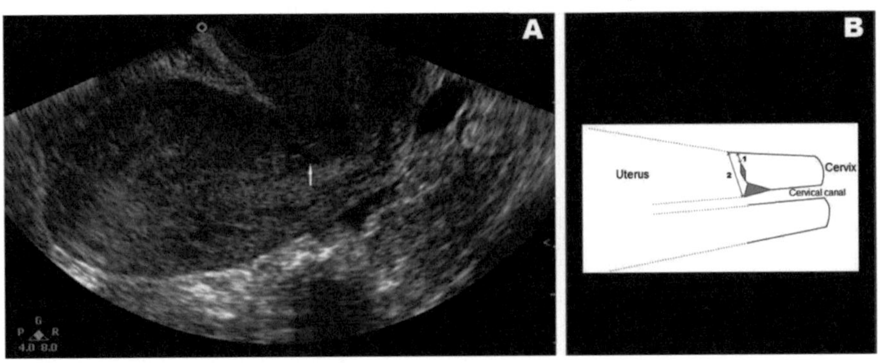

Figure 1.
Cesarean scar defect presented as a hypoechogenic indentation within the myometrium in the LUS (arrow) with ultrasound longitudinal scan of the uterus (A) and measurement of the cesarean scar defect in a schematic drawing (B): Thickness of residual myometrium over the defect (1) and thickness of myometrium adjacent to the defect (2), and the gray shaded areas representing a scar defect. Modified from Au et al. [1].

Variable		Univariate		Multivariate	
		OR (95% CI)	P	OR (95% CI)	P
Cesarean scar	Intact scar*	Reference	—	Reference	—
	Defective scar	3.32 (1.64–6.75)	<0.001	3.34 (1.63–6.83)	<0.001
Parity	1	Reference	—	Reference	—
	≥2	1.19 (0.59–2.41)	0.622	0.82 (0.22–3.07)	0.773
Previous TOP	No	Reference	—	Reference	—
	Yes	1.24 (0.61–2.54)	0.548	1.22 (0.58–2.57)	0.602
Number of previous Cesarean deliveries	1	Reference	—	Reference	—
	≥2	1.18 (0.60–2.35)	0.63	1.36 (0.38–4.88)	0.638

Modified from Au et al. [1]. Data are given as median (interquartile range) or n (%). OR, odds ratio.
**Ratio between the thickness of residual myometrium over the defect and thickness of myometrium adjacent to the defect.*

Table 1.
Association between obstetric factors and failed early termination of pregnancy (TOP) by oral mifepristone and misoprostol in 183 women with previous cesarean delivery.

thickness adjacent to the defect was not significantly different between the groups, but the median of the residual myometrium over the defect was substantially lower in women with failed TOP as compared with those with successful TOP. The median ratio of the thickness of the residual myometrium over the defect of the thickness of the myometrium adjacent to the defect was considerably higher in women with failed TOP as compared with those with successful TOP. Based on these results, Au et al. [1] concluded that women with cesarean scar defects are at increased risk of failed TOP, especially if a defect with the residual myometrial thickness is smaller than one-third of the adjacent myometrial thickness, tended to have a greater chance of the failed TOP.

Lincenberg et al. [2] recently reported a case of extruding a fetal part through the ruptured cesarean scar defect in the lower uterine segment (LUS) in a 28-year-old patient with previous four CSs and presence of a dichorionic diamniotic pregnancy of 10 weeks and 2 days of gestation age (**Figure 2**).

During emergency surgery, the authors removed the exteriorized fetus and saved the remaining fetus in the uterine cavity. Then, they repaired the ruptured scar defect in the LUS with a single layer running-locking suture with good hemostasis. This pregnancy was prolonged up to 23 weeks, an emergency CS was performed by a classical uterine incision and the fetus was delivered together with the placenta. The remaining piece of placenta was removed from the anterior LUS with Banjo curettage. The uterine incision was sutured and good hemostasis was achieved. The postoperative period was complicated by acute blood loss followed by blood transfusion. The patient recovered well and was discharged home in good condition on postoperative day 3 [2].

Analogous case of surgical management of a heterotopic cesarean scar pregnancy with preservation of an intrauterine pregnancy was described by Vetter et al. [3]. A 29-year-old pregnant woman was admitted at 5 weeks of gestational age (WGA) with mild discharge as a spot. Ultrasound revealed a heterotopic cesarean scar pregnancy. The patient underwent resection of the ectopic pregnancy through

Parameters		Successful TOP (n = 36)	Failed TOP (n = 23)	P
Width of defect (mm)		3.4 (1.50–5.50)	3.2 (2.10–4.50)	0.363†
Depth of defect (mm)		8.4 (4.35–10.30)	10.4 (7.60–13.50)	0.035†
Residual myometrium over defect (mm)		6.4 (4.20–10.70)	3.4 (1.80–6.80)	0.017†
Myometrial thickness adjacent to defect (mm)		15.3 (13.80–16.15)	15.2 (13.30–15.80)	0.610†
Myometrial thickness ratio (%)*		58.5 (32.4–73.6)	75.0 (55.8–88.5)	0.014†
Ratio*	<30%	12 (33.3)	16 (69.6)	0.023‡
	30–70%	15 (41.7)	5 (21.7)	
	>70%	9 (25.0)	2 (8.7)	

*Modified from Au et al. [1]. Data are given as median (interquartile range) or n (%).*Ratio between the thickness of residual myometrium over the defect and thickness of myometrium adjacent to the defect.*
†Mann-Whitney U-test.
‡Chi-square test.

Table 2.
Cesarean scar defect size in 59 women with previous cesarean delivery and CSD at transvaginal ultrasound who received oral mifepristone and misoprostol for early termination of pregnancy (TOP), according to whether TOP was successful or failed.

mini-laparotomy with the preservation of an intrauterine pregnancy, which resulted in the delivery of a pre-term baby [3].

Naji et al. [4] evaluated the cesarean scar changes longitudinally throughout the pregnancy to relate the initial scar measurements (**Figure 3**). These findings were incorporated with demographic and obstetric variables, as well as with final pregnancy outcomes. LUS was assessed by using real-time ultrasound to identify the cesarean scar defects. Two components of the cesarean scars were identified: a hypoechoic part or "apparent defect" and any residual myometrium located above the scar defect expressed as the residual myometrial thickness for measurement purposes as (A) width of hypoechoic part, (B) depth of hypoechoic part, (C) residual myometrial thickness, (D) utero-vesical fold, and (E) internal Cervical Os [4].

The prospective observational study by Naji et al. [4] included 320 patients in total, among them 284 patients with visible scars and 36 women with nonvisible scars. There were 153 and 14 patients with two CSs among the women with visible and nonvisible scars, respectively, whereas 131 and 22 patients experienced only one CS among the women with visible and non-visible scars, respectively. While analyzing the changes of the cesarean scar size throughout pregnancy, Naji et al. [4] found the average increase of 1.8 (95% CI, 1.7–1.9) mm in the width of the hypoechoic part of the scar per trimester (**Table 3**), whereas the depth and length of the hypoechoic part decreased over time, with an average decrease of 1.8 (95% CI, 1.7–1.9) mm and 1.9 (95% CI, 1.8–2.0) mm per trimester, respectively. RMT decreased by an average of 1.1 (95% CI, 1.0–1.2) mm per trimester. These changes were clear in a mixed modeling analysis of the cesarean scar disturbances over time (**Figure 4**).

Naji et al. [4] reported two cases of a cesarean scar rupture among their study population. They also found that the decrease in the residual myometrial thickness (RMT) between the first and second trimester was 2.7 and 2.5 mm, respectively, in those patients with cesarean scar ruptures. An average RMT in these cases was

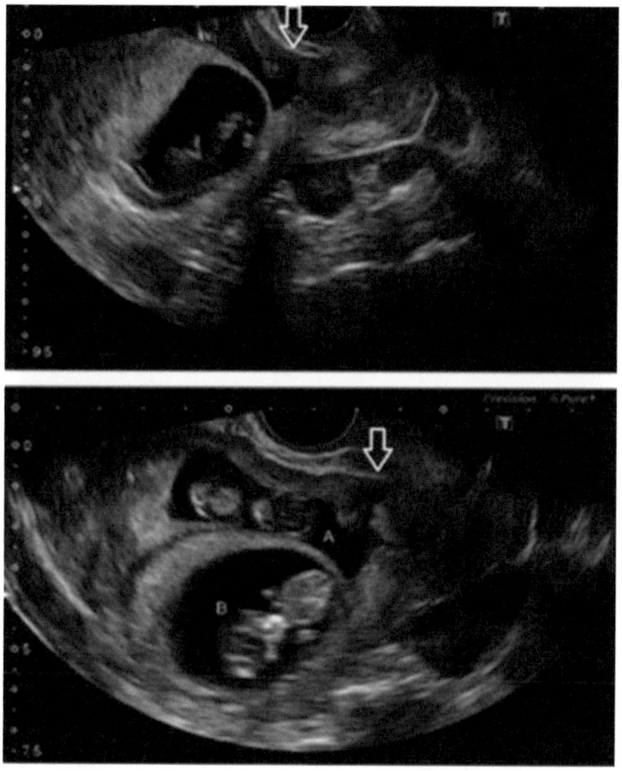

Figure 2.
The arrows are used to demonstrate the cesarean scar in the LUS, into which implanted twin (A). Modified from Lincenberg et al. [2].

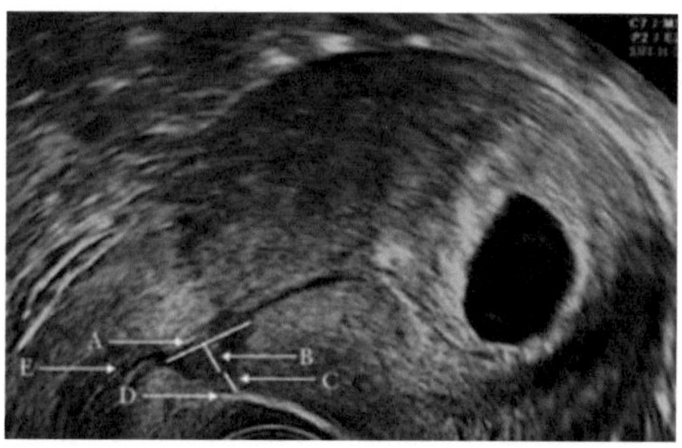

Figure 3.
Sagittal ultrasound image showing anatomical location of features measured to quantify the size of component parts of cesarean scar defects by using TVS in the first trimester of pregnancy. A-width of hypoechoic part; B-depth of hypoechoic part; C-residual myometrial thickness; D-uterovesical fold; E-internal cervical os. Modified from Naji et al. [4].

0.5 mm at the second trimester scan, as compared to 3.6 mm for the other cases [4]. Based on the obtained clinical results and their mixed model analysis, Naji et al. [4] concluded that the changes of cesarean scar dimensions throughout pregnancy and cesarean scar rupture were associated with a smaller residual myometrial thickness and a greater decrease in this parameter during pregnancy. They also suggested that there is a potential to test absolute values and observed alterations in cesarean scar measurements as predictors of uterine scar rupture or vaginal birth after cesarean (VBAC) trial outcome [4].

Scar characteristic	Trimester 1	Trimester 2	Trimester 3	P*
Scar width (mm)	3.6 (3.0–4.7)	5.3 (4.0–6.6)	7.4 (6.1–8.9)	0.0001
Scar depth (mm)	8.3 (6.6–10.2)	6.2 (5.1–7.5)	4.8 (3.7–5.6)	0.0001
Scar length (mm)	10.4 (8.6–12.7)	8.0 (7.2–9.9)	6.8 (5.9–8.1)	0.0001
RMT (mm)	5.3 (4.7–6.2)	3.5 (2.8–4.2)	3.5 (2.5–3.6)	0.0001

Data are shown as median (interquartile range). RMT, residual myometrial thickness; False discovery rate. Modified from Naji et al. [4].
**One-way repeated-measures ANOVA.*

Table 3.
Cesarean scar size and dimensions in each trimester of pregnancy.

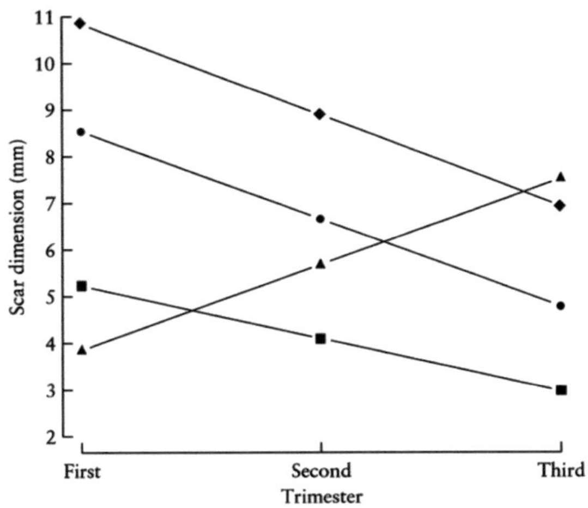

Figure 4.
Mean scar dimensions according to trimester, relating to the fitted fixed effects from mixed-effects modeling. Modified from Naji et al. (2013). Diamond, residual myometrial thickness; Circle, scar depth; Square, scar length; Triangle, scar width.

Xiaoxia et al. [5] analyzed 67 cases of uterine rupture out of 128,599 deliveries in a single-center retrospective study in China. Uterine wall ruptures were found in 88.0% of cases (59/67). They found cesarean scar spontaneous incomplete ruptures in 52 cases, which were repaired without maternal and fetal complications. Emergency rescue operations were performed in 15 cases because of fetal distress or death, severe acute abdomen, prepartum or postpartum vaginal bleeding, maternal hypovolemia, and 12 perinatal fetal deaths. Among them, the uterine rupture was diagnosed with a history of clinical symptoms and signs in 6/15 cases. Ultrasound showed a dead fetus in the peritoneal cavity in 3/15 cases before the exploratory LT, while during LT a dead fetus was found in 6/15 cases in the abdomen. The uterus was preserved in 5/15 cases and hysterectomy took place in 10/15 cases [5]. The authors concluded that a previous cesarean scar became the leading cause of uterine rupture among other surgical procedures, such as assisted delivery operations, intrauterine manipulations and surgical treatment of large myomas and uterine malformations.

The most important issue related with cesarean scar pregnancies is the possibility of uterine rupture, especially in cases of VBAC. Subsequently, in the 1980s, ultrasound was applied to diagnose scar defects following CS [6, 7]. Václavinková and Westin [6] in a retrospective study of 2542 cases found 11.3% CS rate. Among them, 2.8% cesarean scars exhibited deficient healing.

The authors found smooth or pathologically deformed structures corresponding to the cesarean scar region [6, 7]. Further 68 women were under more detailed prospective examination, and the authors observed a uterine scar rupture in two patients. They concluded that the sensitivity of the ultrasonic method was 67% and the specificity 96% in the diagnosis of cesarean scar healing disturbances [6]. Bedi et al. [7] reported that ultrasound examination was able to diagnose uterine rupture by demonstrating intra- or extraperitoneal hematoma in the correct clinical setting.

Fukuda et al. [8] assessed LUS thickness perioperatively in 35 women with previous CS and in 29 women without CS who were subjected to elective CS before the labor. LUS thickness was assessed immediately before CS by ultrasound and intraoperatively by ophthalmic calipers before delivery of the fetus, and surgeons were asked to classify the thickness of LUS according to the Grade system (**Table 4**). Fukuda et al. [8] found complete dehiscence of the scar in three cases (8.6%), thin LUS in 4 cases (11.4%) and no scar defect in 28 cases (80.0%) among 35 women with previous CS. The authors demonstrated correlations between LUS thickness assessed by ultrasound prior to CS and intraoperative ophthalmic caliper measurements before and immediately after delivery, as well as results of visual grading by surgeons [8].

Michaels et al. [9] examined 58 high-risk patients to diagnose cesarean scar defects in the LUS. These patients delivered by CS, and 12 nulliparous women with no risk were used as control. The authors found cesarean scar defects in 20.7% (12/58) cases among high-risk women who experienced CS. The positive and negative predictive values were 92.3 and 100%, respectively.

Uterine scar dehiscence can happen, especially, in cases of a very short interval between pregnancies. The repeated ultrasound performed during

Characteristics of women and grades	N	LUS thickness before		Correlation coefficient and p-value	LUS thickness fetus delivery (ophthalmic calipers, mm)
		CS (US, mm)	Fetus delivery (ophthalmic calipers, mm)		
Women without previous CS	29	2.7 ± 0.6	2.7 ± 0.6	r = 0.980 P < 0.001	4.4 ± 1.1 (n = 11)
Women with previous CS					
Overall	35	1.9 ± 0.9	1.8 ± 0.9	r = 0.985 P < 0.001	3.4 ± 1.1 (n = 17)
Grade I: neither thinning nor loss of continuity of the LUS – no scar defect	28	2.2 ± 0.7	2.1 ± 0.8	R = 0.970 <0.001	3.7 ± 0.9 (n = 14)
Grade II: thinning and/or loss of continuity of the LUS but fetal hair not visible – thin LUS	4	1.0 ± 0.2	0.8 ± 0.1	R = 0.707 =0.29	2.4 ± 0.1 (n = 2)
Grade III: thinning or absence of the LUS and fetal hair visible – complete dehiscence of the scar	3	0.4 ± 0.1	0.4 ± 0.1	R = 0.866 =0.33	1.1 (n = 1)

Modified from CS Fukuda et al. [13].

Table 4.
LUS thickness immediately before, during and after.

pregnancy can help to define the cesarean scar dehiscence in women with previous CS. Supplementation of the above-presented case reports by the systematic review of the LUS measurements performed between 35 and 40 WGA by Jastrow et al. [10] can improve our understanding. In this study uterine rupture and uterine scar dehiscence diagnosed during CS in 1834 women were extracted from 12 studies. One study was an exception, when a pelvic bimanual revision of the LUS was performed after delivery to diagnose uterine scar dehiscence. Thus, cesarean scar defects were identified among the women subjected to VBAC and CSs. The authors demonstrated that the weighted mean difference with (95% CI) was 0.98 mm (0.37–1.59 mm) for the thinner full LUS, and 1.13 mm (0.32–1.94 mm) for thinner myometrial layer in the women with uterine scar defects. Further, additional summary receiver operating characteristic (SROC) analysis and summary diagnostic odds ratios were used to evaluate and compare the area under the curve and the association between the LUS thickness and uterine scar defect. Subsequently, the SROC analysis revealed a stronger association between the full LUS thickness and uterine scar defect than the association between myometrial layer thickness and scar defect [10].

The characteristics of the ultrasound studies examining the full LUS thickness were additionally analyzed, taking into account the predicting value of TAS [11–15] and TVS [16, 17] ultrasound approaches for cesarean scar defects (**Table 5**).

Although the authors included the data by Bujold et al. [18] into the TA subgroup, we excluded this study from our analysis.

Our supplementary analysis of these results showed that scar defects were registered in 6.1% (64/1051) and in 14.4% (19/132) cases by TA and TV, respectively, during ultrasound examinations of full LUS thickness before delivery. According to this analysis, there was a higher rate of cesarean scar defects after examining the full LUS thickness by the TV approach, as compared to the TA ultrasound (see **Table 5**).

Then, the characteristics of ultrasound studies that examined the myometrial layer of the LUS, were also re-analyzed, taking into account the predicting

References	SA/SS (n)	BSR	TOL (n)	VBAC, n	CS, n	SD, n (%)	total, n
1. Fukuda et al. [13]	TA/84	No	NA	24	60	5 (6.0)	84
2. Rozenberg et al. [11]	TA/642	Yes	517	386	256	25 (3.9)	642
3. Tanik et al. [14]	TA/50	No	0	0	50	23 (46.0)	50
4. Rozenberg et al. [12]	TA/198	No	170	131	62	2 (1.0)	192
5. Suzuki et al. [15]	TA/83#	No	44	27	56	9 (10.8)	83
6. Montanari et al. [16]	TV/61	Yes	NA	8	53	17 (27.9)	61
7. Sen et al. [17]	TV/71*	Yes	52	33	38	2 (2.8)	71
Total	TA-1293	Yes −1	856	658	630	64 (6.0)	1051
	TV-132	Yes −2	52	41	91	19 (14.4)	132

LUS, lower uterine segment; SA, ultrasound approach; SS, sample size; BSR, blinded sonographic results; TOL, trial of labor; VBAC, vaginal birth after cesarean section; CS, cesarean section; SD, scar defect; TA, transabdominal; TV, transvaginal; $, number of VBAC and CSs; &, incorporated into total TA or TV approaches.

Table 5.
Characteristics of the ultrasound studies examined full LUS thickness.

value of TA [19–21] and TV [18, 22] ultrasound approaches for cesarean scar defects (**Table 6**).

Moreover scar defects were registered in 7.9% (28/356) and in 3.5% (10/289) cases after evaluating the myometrial layer of the LUS before delivery by TA and TV ultrasound, respectively (see **Table 6**). According to these results, there was a higher rate of scar defects after evaluation of the myometrial layer of the LUS before delivery by TA, as compared to TV ultrasound.

The authors demonstrated the optimal cut-off value, which varied from 2.0 to 3.5 mm, for the full LUS thickness (**Figure 5A**), and from 1.4 to 2.0 mm for a myometrial layer (**Figure 5B**). However, the authors concluded that at present there is not an ideal cut-off value to be recommended, taking into account the requirements for more standardized measurement methods.

References	SA/SS (n)	BSR	TOL, n	VBAC, n$	CS, n$	SD, n (%)	Total, n$
1. Asakura et al. [19]	TA/186	Yes	132	63	123	9 (4.8)	186
2. Gotoh et al. [20]	TA/68	No	0	0	68	17 (25.0)	68
3. Cheung et al. [21]	TA/102*	No	50	32	70	2 (2.0)	102
4. Bujold et al. [18]	TV/223	No	125	90	146	9 (3.8)	236
5. Cheung et al. [22]	TV/53	No	28	18	35	1 (1.9)	53
Total	TA-356	Yes –1	182	95	261	28 (7.9)	356
	TV-276	Yes –0	153	108	181	10 (3.5)	289

LUS, lower uterine segment; SA, ultrasound approach; SS, sample size; BSR, blinded sonographic results; TOL, trial of labor; VBAC, vaginal birth after cesarean section; CS, cesarean section; SD, scar defect; TA, transabdominal; TV, transvaginal; $, number of VBAC and CSs; &, incorporated into total TA or TV approaches. *LUS appearance described only for CSs.*

Table 6.
Characteristics of ultrasound studies examining the myometrial layer of the LUS.

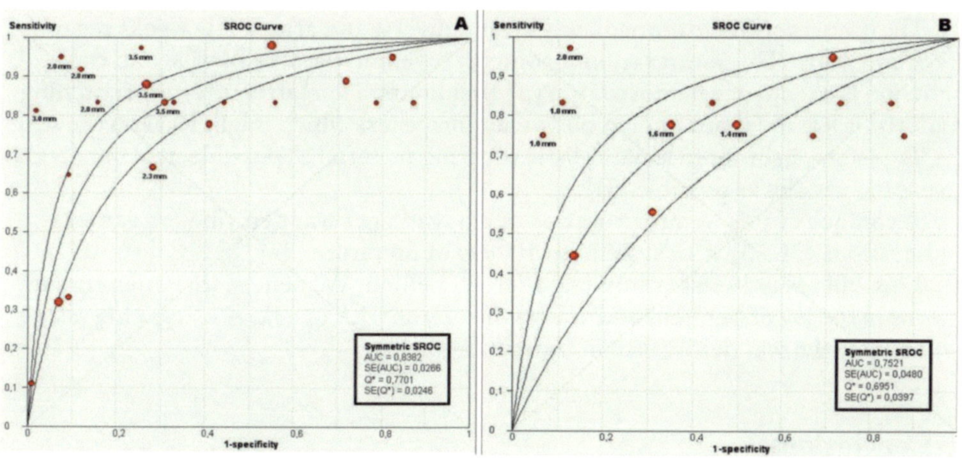

Figure 5.
Summary receiver operating characteristic curve analyses of the association between: Full LUS thickness and the risk of uterine scar defect (A); Myometrial thickness and the risk of uterine scar defect (B).

3. Discussion

Today Cragin's opinion "once a Caesarean, always a Caesarean" [23] is proved by highly increasing CS rate worldwide.

In the last decades, the number of Cesarean Sections increased steadily [24]. One of the reasons is the promoting of Cesarean Section by request of the mother [25].

As a result, more placental implantation pathologies occur [26], and certainly more problems related to scar dehiscence following repeated pregnancies following Cesarean Sections.

The best way to prevent these complications is certainly by reducing the number of Cesarean Sections, mainly at low-risk pregnancies. In our group, it was successfully achieved by asking for a documented second opinion for each non-emergency Cesarean Section.

When a Cesarean Section is done, it is important to perform the operation in a way that the full thickness of the uterine wall, as well as its strength, will be preserved.

It is important to analyze what are the reasons for uterine wall defects and how are they related to the surgical method.

It was shown by Di Spiezio et al. that one or two layers suturing of the uterine wall do not make any difference concerning the incidence of Cesarean scar defects as well as the uterine dehiscence and rate of ruptures in subsequent pregnancies [27].

Although a second layer did not show any benefit concerning the thickness of the uterine wall [28].

If one or two layers of sutures are not the etiology of dehiscence in subsequent pregnancies, it is important to analyze the relevant reason.

It is known that sutured muscle tissue will never regain its original strength, in contrary to fibrous tissue. Therefore, the less muscle tissue to be cut the better are the chances for a stronger scar.

Rorie analyzed the histological structure of the uterus and found out that the amount of smooth muscle in the upper third of the cervix is 28%, and in the body of the uterus 68.8% [29].

It means the lower the incision in the uterus, the less damage to the uterine wall.

As a result, it is important to incise the urine bladder plica, push the bladder down, and cut the uterine wall as low as possible. This is in contrary to the nowadays practice to open the uterus above the plica [30].

The uterus contracts immediately after delivery, and after a few weeks regains its original size. The sutures cannot contract together with the uterus, and their function is to enhance hemostasis in the first hours. Thereafter, the more stitching material is left the more foreign body reaction occurs which might weaken the scar.

Therefore, in order to leave as little suturing material as possible, it is important to use big needles as possible [31].

Technique of this Cesarean section and advantages was described in earlier publications [31–36] with systematic review of literature [37].

This will result in less suture material left behind. We believe that opening the uterus in the lower segment and suture the uterus with one layer using a big needle will reduce the scar dehiscence in future pregnancies.

4. Conclusions

The cesarean scar is a significant risk factor for the following pregnancies and especially deliveries. In this chapter, we discussed the diagnosis, incidence, detection, manifestations, and prognosis of pregnancy and delivery with cesarean scars.

A systematic review of current literature showed that a manifestation of cesarean scars during the following pregnancies is not predictable, in general, although modern visualization technologies could reveal some specific features of scar defects that are associated with complications during pregnancy and delivery. However, there is no factor, which could serve as the main prognostic guide for obstetricians to make a decision for VBAC, thus Edwin Cragin's phrase "once a cesarean, always a cesarean" has represented the essential health care issue over the century. At the moment, the most reasonable measurements to prevent uterine scar complications are reducing the rate of Cesarean Sections, opening the uterus transversely in the lower segment, and stitching the uterus with one layer only continuously using a big needle preferable by Stark technique of Cesarean section.

Acknowledgements

The authors would like to sincerely thank Mrs. Maya A. Bessarabova for her inestimable assistance of the manuscript preparation.

Conflict of interest

No conflict of interest exists.

Author details

Ospan Mynbaev[1,2], Ioannis Kosmas[3], Zhongjie Shi[1,4*], Sergei Firichenko[1,5], Avinoam Tzabari[1,2,6], Lin Ma[1,7], Leila Kindarova[8], Tatiana Babenko[1,9], Styliani Salta[2,10], Antonio Malvasi[1,2], Ivano Raimondo[2,11], Andrea Tinelli[1,12], Victor Gomel[1,13] and Michael Stark[1,2,14,15]

1 The International Bureau of Human Body Design, Biomodeling, and Biosensoring, Moscow Institute of Physics and Technology (State University), Moscow, Russia

2 The New European Surgical Academy, Berlin, Germany

3 Ioannina University, Ioannina, Greece

4 Wayne State University, Detroit, USA

5 Moscow State University of Medicine and Dentistry, Moscow, Russia

6 Emergency Obstetrics and Gynecologic Unit, Mayanei Hayeshua Medical Center, Bnei Brak, Israel

7 Henry Ford Hospital, Detroit, USA

8 Russian-German Center of Reproduction and Clinical Embryology "Generation NEXT", Moscow, Russia

9 City Clinical Hospital for Emergency Medical Services N4, Stavropol Krai, Russia

10 Haemophilia Centre, University Hospitals of Leicester, Leicester, UK

11 Gynecologic and Obstetric Clinic, Sassari University, Sassari, Italy

12 Division of Experimental Endoscopic Surgery, Imaging, Technology and Minimally Invasive Therapy, Department of Obstetrics and Gynecology, Vito Fazzi Hospital, Lecce, Italy

13 Department of Obstetrics and Gynecology, Women's Hospital, University of British Columbia, Vancouver, BC, Canada

14 Department of Gynecological Oncology, Berlin Humboldt University Hospital Charite, Berlin, Germany

15 The ELSAN Group, Paris, France

*Address all correspondence to: zshi@med.wayne.edu

References

[1] Au HK, Liu CF, Tzeng CR, Chien LW. Association between ultrasonographic parameters of cesarean scar defect and outcome of early termination of pregnancy. Ultrasound in Obstetrics & Gynecology. 2016;**47**:506-510. DOI: 10.1002/uog.14877

[2] Lincenberg KR, Behrman ER, Bembry JS, Kovac CM. Uterine rupture with cesarean scar heterotopic pregnancy with survival of the intrauterine twin. Case Reports in Obstetrics and Gynecology. 2016;**2016**:6832094. DOI: 10.1155/2016/6832094

[3] Vetter MH, Andrzejewski J, Murnane A, Lang C. Surgical management of a heterotopic cesarean scar pregnancy with preservation of an intrauterine pregnancy. Obstetrics and Gynecology. 2016;**128**:613-616. DOI: 10.1097/AOG.0000000000001514

[4] Naji O, Daemen A, Smith A, Abdallah Y, Saso S, Stalder C, et al. Changes in cesarean section scar dimensions during pregnancy: A prospective longitudinal study. Ultrasound in Obstetrics & Gynecology. 2013;**41**:556-562. DOI: 10.1002/uog.12334

[5] Xiaoxia B, Zhengping W, Xiaofu Y. Clinical study on 67 cases with uterine rupture. Zhonghua Fu Chan Ke Za Zhi. 2014;**49**:331-335

[6] Václavinková V, Westin B. Ultrasonic diagnosis of scar defects following cesarean section. Zentralblatt für Gynäkologie. 1984;**106**(10):686-692

[7] Bedi DG, Salmon A, Winsett MZ, Fagan CJ, Kumar R. Ruptured uterus: Sonographic diagnosis. Journal of Clinical Ultrasound. 1986;**14**:529-533

[8] Fukuda M, Fukuda K, Shimizu T, Bujold E. Ultrasound assessment of lower uterine segment thickness during pregnancy, labour, and the postpartum period. Journal of Obstetrics and Gynaecology Canada. 2016;**38**:134-140. DOI: 10.1016/j.jogc.2015.12.009

[9] Michaels WH, Thompson HO, Boutt A, Schreiber FR, Michaels SL, Karo J. Ultrasound diagnosis of defects in the scarred lower uterine segment during pregnancy. Obstetrics and Gynecology. 1988;**71**:112-120

[10] Jastrow N, Chaillet N, Roberge S, Morency AM, Lacasse Y, Bujold E. Sonographic lower uterine segment thickness and risk of uterine scar defect: A systematic review. Journal of Obstetrics and Gynaecology Canada. 2010;**32**:321-327. DOI: 10.1016/S1701-2163(16)34475-9

[11] Rozenberg P, Goffinet F, Phillippe HJ, Nisand I. Ultrasonographic measurement of lower uterine segment to assess risk of defects of scarred uterus. Lancet. 1996;**347**:281-284

[12] Rozenberg P, Goffinet F, Philippe HJ, Nisand I. Thickness of the lower uterine segment: Its influence in the management of patients with previous cesarean sections. European Journal of Obstetrics, Gynecology, and Reproductive Biology. 1999;**87**:39-45

[13] Fukuda M, Fukuda K, Mochizuki M. Examination of previous caesarean section scars by ultrasound. Archives of Gynecology and Obstetrics. 1988;**243**:221-224

[14] Tanik A, Ustun C, Cil E, Arslan A. Sonographic evaluation of the wall thickness of the lower uterine segment in patients with previous cesarean section. Journal of Clinical Ultrasound. 1996;**24**:355-357

[15] Suzuki S, Sawa R, Yoneyama Y, Asakura H, Araki T. Preoperative diagnosis of dehiscence of the lower

uterine segment in patients with a single previous caesarean section. The Australian & New Zealand Journal of Obstetrics & Gynaecology. 2000;**40**:402-404

[16] Montanari L, Alfei A, Drovanti A, Lepadatu C, Lorenzi D, Facchini D, et al. Transvaginal ultrasonic evaluation of the thickness of the section of the uterine wall in previous cesarean sections [article in Italian]. Minerva Ginecologica. 1999;**51**:107-112

[17] Sen S, Malik S, Salhan S. Ultrasonographic evaluation of lower uterine segment thickness in patients of previous cesarean section. International Journal of Gynecology & Obstetrics. 2004;**87**:215-219

[18] Bujold E, Jastrow N, Simoneau J, Brunet S, Gauthier RJ. Prediction of complete uterine rupture by sonographic evaluation of the lower uterine segment. American Journal of Obstetrics and Gynecology. 2009;**201**:320.e1-320.e6. DOI: 10.1016/j.ajog.2009.06.014

[19] Asakura H, Nakai A, Ishikawa G, Suzuki S, Araki T. Prediction of uterine dehiscence by measuring lower uterine segment thickness prior to the onset of labor: Evaluation by transvaginal ultrasonography. Journal of Nippon Medical School. 2000;**67**:352-356

[20] Gotoh H, Masuzaki H, Yoshida A, Yoshimura S, Miyamura T, Ishimaru T. Predicting incomplete uterine rupture with vaginal sonography during the late second trimester in women with prior cesarean. Obstetrics and Gynecology. 2000;**95**:596-600

[21] Cheung VY. Sonographic measurement of the lower uterine segment thickness in women with previous caesarean section. Journal of Obstetrics and Gynaecology Canada. 2005;**27**:674-681

[22] Cheung VY, Constantinescu OC, Ahluwalia BS. Sonographic evaluation of the lower uterine segment in patients with previous cesarean delivery. Journal of Ultrasound in Medicine. 2004;**23**:1441-1447

[23] Cragin EB. Conservatism in obstetrics. The New York Medical Journal. 1916;**104**:1-3

[24] Barber EL, Lundsberg LS, Belanger K, et al. Indications contributing to the increasing cesarean delivery rate. Obstetrics and Gynecology. 2011;**118**(1):29-38

[25] Husslein P, Wertaschnigg D. Elective cesarean section--delivery mode of the future or social misconception? Therapeutische Umschau. 2002;**59**(12):660-666

[26] El Gelany S, Mosbeh MH, Ibrahim EM, et al. Placenta Accreta Spectrum (PAS) disorders: Incidence, risk factors and outcomes of different management strategies in a tertiary referral hospital in Minia, Egypt: A prospective study. BMC Pregnancy and Childbirth. 2019;**19**(1):313

[27] Di Spiezio Sardo A, Saccone G, McCurdy R, et al. Risk of cesarean scar defect following single- vs double-layer uterine closure: Systematic review and meta-analysis of randomized controlled trials. Ultrasound in Obstetrics & Gynecology. 2017;**50**(5):578-583

[28] Bennich G, Rudnicki M, Wilken-Jensen C, et al. Impact of adding a second-layer to a single unlocked closure of cesarean uterine incision: A randomized controlled trial. Ultrasound in Obstetrics & Gynecology. 2016;**47**(4):417-422

[29] Rorie DK, Newton M. Histologic and chemical studies of the smooth muscle in the human cervix and uterus. American Journal of Obstetrics and Gynecology. 1967;**99**(4):466-469

[30] O'Neill HA, Egan G, Walsh CA, et al. Omission of the bladder flap at caesarean section reduces delivery time without increased morbidity: A meta-analysis of randomised controlled trials. European Journal of Obstetrics, Gynecology, and Reproductive Biology. 2014;**174**:20-26

[31] Stark M. Does size matter? Journal Of The Turkish-German Gynecological Association. 2016;**17**(3):175

[32] Stark M, Chavkin Y, Kupfersztain C, Guedj P, Finkel AR. Evaluation of combinations of procedures in cesarean section. International Journal of Gynaecology and Obstetrics. 1995;**48**(3):273-276

[33] Holmgren G, Sjöholm L. The Misgav Ladach method of caesarean section: Evolved by Joel-Cohen and Michael Stark in Jerusalem. Tropical Doctor. 1996;**26**(4):150-157

[34] Holmgren G, Sjöholm L, Stark M. The Misgav Ladach method for cesarean section: Method description. Acta Obstetricia et Gynecologica Scandinavica. 1999;**78**(7):615-621

[35] Stark M. Clinical evidence that suturing the peritoneum after laparotomy is unnecessary for healing. World Journal of Surgery. 1993;**17**(3):419

[36] Stark M. In the era of 'non-closure of the peritoneum', how to open it? (not every simple method is optimal, but every optimal method is simple). Acta Obstetricia et Gynecologica Scandinavica. 2009;**88**(1):119

[37] Mynbaev O, Babenko TI, Ahmadi F, Raimondo I, Kosmas IP, Mishutina AA, et al. Uterine morbidity: Cesarean section scar complications. In: Tinelli A, Pacheco LA, Haimovich S, editors. Chapter 41 in Hysteroscopy. Cham: Springer; 2018. pp. 421-468. DOI: 10.1007/978-3-319-57559-9_41

Chapter 5

Obesity: Unique Challenges at the Time of Cesarean Delivery

Kristina Roloff, Suzanne Cao, Camille Okekpe, Inessa Dombrovsky and Guillermo Valenzuela

Abstract

The obesity epidemic has touched all aspects of obstetric care, including the practice of cesarean delivery. Obesity is an independent risk factor for cesarean delivery, and the increased prevalence of obesity has contributed to the overall rise in primary cesarean delivery seen over the past few decades. Because of the frequent existence of co-morbidities such as hypertension and diabetes, obesity is a plausible contributor to rising maternal mortality. In addition, obese women who undergo both primary and repeat cesarean delivery have a higher chance to develop surgical and post-operative complications, including wound infection and thromboembolic events. Surgical complications increase steadily with increasing maternal weight. In this chapter, we will review the incidence and contributing factors that lead to cesarean delivery in obese patients, peri-operative complications, and strategies to reduce these risks in obese women undergoing cesarean delivery.

Keywords: cesarean delivery, obesity, super-obesity

1. Introduction

Cecelia presents for a routine new obstetric appointment for her second pregnancy. She has had one prior pregnancy, and does not identify any health problems on her intake paperwork. However, she is markedly obese, and her weight is in excess of 500 pounds, more than the average in-office scale can measure. Adequate understanding of risks and management strategies to mitigate her risk is needed to optimize the chances of a health pregnancy outcome.

The prevalence of obesity, defined as body mass index (BMI) ≥ 30 kg/m^2, and super-obesity (BMI ≥ 50 kg/m^2) is on the rise in reproductive aged women. Pregnancy complications such as gestational diabetes, preeclampsia, macrosomia, and stillbirth are more common in obese women than in normal weight patients. Many of these complications occur in a dose dependent fashion; the higher the BMI category, the more likely complications are to occur. The obese patient has both an increased risk for needing an indicated primary cesarean delivery, an increased risk for peri-operative complications, and is at higher risk for failed trial of labor after cesarean delivery. The super-obese patient, in particular, presents a unique challenge to obstetricians planning and preparing for cesarean delivery.

In this chapter, we will review the evidence of surgical risk at the time of cesarean delivery, management options to reduce surgical risks, and practical considerations in performing a cesarean delivery in the obese parturient.

IntechOpen

2. Incidence of cesarean delivery in obese women

Estimates of primary cesarean delivery rates in obese patients undergoing trial of labor range from 23 to 49%, and increase with increasing maternal BMI (23–46% BMI $\geq$30 kg/m^2, 30–47% BMI $\geq$ 40 kg/m^2, 45–49% BMI $\geq$ 50 kg/m^2) [1–5]. The most common indications for cesarean delivery are labor arrest (61%) and non-reassuring fetal status (28%) [1]. Pre-labor primary cesarean delivery also increases with increasing BMI class [5].

3. Factors contributing to cesarean delivery in obese women

The reason for the increased incidence of cesarean delivery in obese women is likely multifactorial, and includes higher chances of macrosomia – and hence labor dystocia, disordered and dysfunctional labor patterns, and provider level responses or bias towards cesarean delivery [5].

The combination of obesity and macrosomia significantly increases the chance of cesarean delivery [6]. Both pre-pregnancy BMI category and gestational weight gain are independent contributors to the development of a large for gestational age or macrosomic infant [7–8]. Obese women tend to have higher gestational weight gain, despite stricter weight gain recommendations, and hence larger birth weight babies [7]. A large fetus, for obvious reasons, predisposes the mother to a protracted labor course and cephalopelvic disproportion leading to an indicated cesarean delivery. In addition, fear of shoulder dystocia and neonatal brachial plexus injury, which occurs more often at delivery of obese women even with lower fetal birth weight, may influence the decision to proceed with cesarean delivery [9]. Because of the chances of fetal macrosomia with advancing gestational age, a strategy of elective induction at term may help to reduce the chances of macrosomia, and hence cesarean delivery. Elective induction was not associated with an increased risk of cesarean delivery in women with BMI $\geq$ 40 kg/m^2 [10].

Obese women also have dysfunctional labor patterns [11]. Obese women are less likely to have spontaneous onset of labor, less likely to achieve vaginal birth following spontaneous labor, and have a higher chance of being exposed to oxytocin than non-obese women [12]. Obese women may require larger doses of oxytocin than their normal weight counterparts, especially when undergoing induction of labor [13]. The pathophysiology of the increased oxytocin requirements and protracted labor course is poorly understood, but may be due to decreased myometrial receptor expression, prostaglandin insensitivity, and impaired myocyte contractility [14]. The dysfunctional and apparently disrupted myometrial activity may contribute to why we see more unplanned cesarean delivery in obese women.

Provider factors also may contribute to the increase chance of cesarean delivery in obese women [15]. Because the decision-to-incision and decision-to-delivery time interval for emergency cesarean delivery is significantly higher in obese women, a recommendation of cesarean delivery may be made earlier, in order to allow adequate time for surgical preparation [16, 17]. The timing of intervention for non-reassuring fetal heart rate patterns likely contributes to increased unplanned cesarean delivery, as well as pre-labor cesarean deliveries [5, 18]. Obese women with prior cesarean delivery are more likely to decline trial of labor after cesarean, which may be due to individual counseling by obstetric providers [19].

Despite the fact that cesarean delivery is performed more often in obese women, it is still a riskier mode of delivery. Planned cesarean delivery, even in super-obese women (BMI $\geq$ 50 kg/m^2) does not reduce maternal or neonatal morbidity [1].

4. Surgical complications

Important peri-operative complications of cesarean delivery in obese women include wound complications (infection, wound separation), thromboembolic events, and adverse neonatal complications. A history of three or more prior cesarean deliveries further increases the chance of complications such as transfusion, low 1 min Apgar score, and wound complications [20]. The timing of repeat cesarean – unscheduled or planned – may also increase surgical and neonatal risks, especially since obese women are more likely to develop pregnancy complications prompting unscheduled repeat cesarean delivery [21]. Other surgical risks, such as bowel, bladder, or ureteral injury, or broad ligament hematoma, appear to be comparably infrequent in obese and super obese women like in normal and overweight women [22]. Super obesity also increases the chance of maternal ICU admission and length of hospitalization, which is largely driven by maternal co-morbid conditions [23, 24].

4.1 Wound complications

Wound complications – separation and infection, occur in approximately 10% of obese women delivered by cesarean [20, 25–27]. The odds ratio for wound complication in obese women is 1.14–1.65 times normal weight controls, when adjusted for many confounders [25]. There is a marked dose response for wound complications by increasing BMI category, with an odds ratio increase of up to 2.0 for every five-unit increment increase in BMI [28]. Chances of wound infection in super-obese women have been reported as high as 30% [29]. In probably the largest sample reported (38,229 women), wound complications occurred in 14% of women with BMI ≥ 45 kg/m^2 following cesarean delivery [25]. Wound separations in particular are seen more frequently in patients with super obesity [30].

An increase in operative time in women who are obese is also dose dependent on BMI category [17, 27, 31]. Longer operative time is strongly correlated to post-operative infection, and may be a potential modifiable factor to reduce wound complication [32]. Other peri-operative and surgical strategies that may help prevent wound complications, such as pre-operative antibiotics, choice of skin incision, and wound closure type are reviewed in Section 4.4.

4.2 Thromboembolic events

Other than cesarean delivery, obesity is the most common risk factor for a venous thromboembolic event (VTE) in pregnancy [33]. The classic Virchow's triad of hypercoagulability, endothelial injury, and stasis of blood flow leads to the well-established risk of VTE during pregnancy. Obesity itself, regardless of mode of delivery, is a significant risk factor for VTE, with reported risks of 1.7 to 5.3 (odds ratio) above normal weight controls [34–37]. Obese pregnant women have greater risk for pulmonary embolism than deep-vein thrombosis (DVT); the adjusted odds ratio for DVT is 4.4 (95% CI 1.6–11.9) and for pulmonary embolism is 14.9 (95% CI 3.0–74.8) [35]. Like other complications, VTE has a dose–response relationship with increasing BMI category [38].

The exact contribution of the combination of obesity and cesarean delivery to VTEs is difficult to quantify. Immobilization and high BMI have a multiplicative effect on risk for VTE [39]. It is very likely that obesity and cesarean delivery also have multiplicative effects on the chance for VTE. Prevention of VTE during cesarean delivery is discussed in Section 6.5.

4.3 Neonatal outcomes

Neonatal outcomes also appear to be influenced by maternal obesity at cesarean delivery. Neonatal morbidity, including low 5-minute Apgar scores (<7), umbilical cord arterial pH < 7.2, base excess ≤8 mmol/L, and neonatal intensive care unit admissions are seen more often in obese women who undergo cesarean delivery. Hypotension during spinal anesthesia, and prolonged puncture time for regional anesthesia is more pronounced in obese women, and has been shown to cause lower umbilical cord pH in obese women undergoing scheduled cesarean delivery [40, 41]. Women who are super-obese at the time of delivery have a 20% chance of neonatal intensive care unit admission [26]. There is a twofold odds increase of adverse neonatal event (low 5 min Apgar score, cardio-pulmonary resuscitation and ventilator support <24 h, neonatal injury, or transient tachypnea of the newborn, grade 3, 4 intraventricular hemorrhage, necrotizing enterocolitis, seizure, respiratory distress syndrome, hypoxic ischemic encephalopathy, meconium aspiration, ventilator support >2 days, sepsis and/or neonatal death) in women with super obesity compared to their normal weight controls [42]. Despite the tendency towards earlier cesarean delivery, the inherent delays and slower decision-to-incision and incision-to-delivery times involved in moving obese women to the delivery suite, and in getting the baby out when marked fetal distress is evident may contribute to adverse neonatal outcomes in some cases [43]. However, planned cesarean delivery is not protective against these risks, and suggests an underlying poorly understood biologic etiology may be the source of the increase in adverse neonatal outcomes seen in obese women.

5. Preparation for cesarean delivery in the obese patient

Performing a cesarean delivery, primary or repeat, in an obese patient poses certain challenges to the obstetrician and the operative team. These challenges are amplified in the super-obese patient, where maternal weight requires particular preparation for routine surgical issues, such as physical plant or space preparation, and informed consent.

5.1 Physical plant preparation

Hospital equipment is often not designed for super-obese women. Operating tables, delivery beds, and even scales may have an upper limit weight rating that is lower than the weight of a super obese woman [44]. It is reasonable for a labor and delivery hospital unit to prepare a sufficient number of rooms with the equipment needed to safely labor and deliver a super-obese women, based on the characteristics of the population they serve and the number of deliveries performed. Our institution maintains one room capable of laboring a patient in excess of 500 pounds. The bed has a higher weight rating and is wider, and has hydraulics to assist in mobility should a move to the operating room be indicated. The room also has a lift on the ceiling above the labor bed, which has been instrumental for aiding the super-obese woman in positioning – for example to lift a leg during placement of a Foley catheter. The room is stocked with equipment and supplies necessary to care for an obese patient.

Since obese women carry a higher risk for cesarean delivery and up to a 50% chance of emergency cesarean delivery, preparation of an operating room even when trial of labor is attempted is necessary [44, 45]. If a wide operating room bed is not available, two standard 50-cm width tables can be secured together [44, 46].

Transferring the patient from a labor and delivery bed to an operating table and then back to a medical bed or gurney can be difficult and lead to staff injury. Air-assisted mattresses can be placed underneath obese patients to facilitate bed transfers (e.g., Hovermatt®, HoverTech International, Bethlehem, PA, USA). Some of these mattresses can also provide lateral turns to help position patients to prevent aortocaval compression [47].

Practical considerations for preparation of the operating room for scheduled or emergency cesarean of an obese patient should be part of labor and delivery policy. Supplies, such as extra-large blood pressure cuffs, clothing, and large pneumatic compression devices should be available. Consideration of adequate surgical supplies including long instrument trays and accessible self-retaining retractors (see Section 6.3), as well as pre-operative preparation for anesthetic administration (see Section 6.1) may improve patient safety [48]. A checklist for physical plant preparation for cesarean delivery in the obese patient is presented in **Table 1**.

Nursing care requires particular attention to support the delivery of an obese patient. Nurses require knowledge of how to use specialized equipment, how to

Labor and delivery room
Bariatric bed with frame and trapeze (motorized to improve mobility)
Bariatric chair
Hydraulic lift
Air assisted mattress
Continuous positive air pressure (CPAP) equipment
Large or extra-large blood pressure cuffs
Extra-large clothing (gowns, panties)
Extra-large pneumatic compression devices
Extra-large wheelchairs (motorized to improve mobility)
Toilet to exceed 500 lb. capacity
Operating room
Bariatric operating table, or two standard 50-cm width tables strapped together securely
Air assisted mattress
Large or extra-large blood pressure cuffs
Extra-large pneumatic compression devices
Long instrument tray
Large OR strap
Long spinal needles
Difficult airway cart
Emergency cricothyroidotomy kit
Glide scope
Laryngeal mask airway
Video guided laryngoscopes
Adhesive straps / Elastoplast tape for pannus management
Self-retaining retractors (Alexis-O cesarean, Doyen)

Table 1.
Physical plant preparation checklist for labor and cesarean delivery in obese patients.

adapt ergonomics to prevent staff and patient injury, and preparation for known risks in order to safely care for obese patients undergoing planned or unplanned cesarean delivery [44, 48]. It may even be reasonable to increase nurse to patient ratios in some situations [48].

5.2 Informed consent

Informed consent for cesarean is best initiated well before the operative day, because of the known increase chance of cesarean in obese women, as well as the particular risks described in section 4. Informed consent obtained during labor is known to be particularly brief, and it is unlikely that obstetricians are able to adequately counsel obese patients about their specific risks at time of cesarean delivery [49]. Lack of informed consent can reinforce a claim of medical malpractice [50]. Discussion that includes culturally sensitive and tailored review of the patients' beliefs about her weight may help improve the environment and her delivery experience, and perhaps even impact her health outcomes [51]. It may be reasonable to address and document informed consent during her routine obstetric care visits, and/or at time of admission to the hospital, well in advance of the actual surgery.

6. Surgical considerations

Challenges facing the obstetric team do not stop at preparation. The performance of a safe cesarean delivery in an obese patient starts with adequate anesthesia, continues with adaptations of surgical technique, and concludes with optimization of post-operative care.

6.1 Anesthetic considerations

General anesthesia, epidural anesthesia, and combined spinal-epidural anesthesia are all options for pain control during cesarean delivery in the obese patient. The choice of anesthetic largely depends on the indication for cesarean and the condition of the fetus at time of delivery.

Regional anesthesia puncture times for epidural and combined spinal-epidural may be prolonged in the obese patient, and may even contribute to delays in decision to delivery times seen in obese women [31, 52]. There is a higher chance of regional anesthesia failures needing conversion to general anesthesia, and a higher chance of high block during spinal anesthesia necessitating general anesthesia in super obese women (BMI $\geq$ 50 kg/m$^{2)}$) [31, 53]. Still, dose reductions for spinal anesthesia have not been proven beneficial in obese patients [54]. The obese patient is at risk for a higher number of punctures at time of spinal placement, simply due to spinal cord distance from skin [41, 55]. Ultrasound guided regional anesthesia placement has been shown to reduce number of punctures in obese women [56].

The risk of regional anesthesia has to be balanced against the risks of general anesthesia in obese patients, which include an inherent difficult airway, transplacental passage of paralytic or sedating medication, and longer incision to delivery times. Pregnancy itself increases the chance of difficult intubation, and obesity appears to multiply this risk – noted to be as high as 33% [57]. The obese patient is also at risk for aspiration (especially if a difficult intubation is encountered), as well as earlier oxygen desaturation [58].

Surgical positioning with a maternal 10–15 degree left lateral tilt is very important in obese women, as their pannus may compress the aorta or vena cava leading to hypotension [44]. Obese women also experience more relative hypotension during spinal anesthesia [40]. In addition, the displacement of the pannus to allow for the surgical incision can increase the chance of respiratory distress [44].

6.2 Selection of the surgical skin incision

There is insufficient evidence to conclude a particular skin incision is superior in the performance of a cesarean delivery in obese women. Various choices have been reported including vertical supra-umbilical, vertical or transverse infraumbilical, and the traditional Pfannenstiel with taping of the pannus if necessary, see **Figure 1**. Vertical incisions are associated with a higher chance of vertical/classical uterine incision, but a lower chance of low 1 and 5 minute Apgar score in women with BMI ≥ 40 kg/m^2 [59, 60]. A randomized feasibility trial of 91 women showed no difference in clinical outcomes between Pfannenstiel and vertical skin incisions, and suggested a larger study would have a low chance of finding a difference [61].

Surgeon preferences lean towards a Pfannenstiel skin incision. A study of surgeon preference of incision type on obese patients between Pfannenstiel with or without taping of the Pannus, and vertical in both emergent and non-emergent cesarean delivery, showed the majority preferred Pfannenstiel with taping of the pannus in both cases [62]. Women prioritize safety when it comes to choice of skin incision. A survey of women with BMI ≥ 40 kg/m^2 showed that neonatal and maternal safety ranked higher in priority over cosmetic outcomes in selection of skin incision [63].

Since a superior skin incision has not been clearly shown, it seems reasonable to choose the skin incision based on clinical characteristics of the maternal habitus, and surgeon preference. If a low vertical, or high transverse skin incision is selected in patients with a pannus, care must be taken to ensure the pannus is not transected.

6.3 Surgical techniques unique to obese women

Barrier self-retaining retractors, such as the Doyen or Alexis-O retractor shown in **Figure 2**, may be used to facilitate exposure and reduce the need for additional hands in surgery to provide retraction. This may be particularly helpful in women with a large pannus. The Hook and Doyen retractor apparatus uses hooks and an

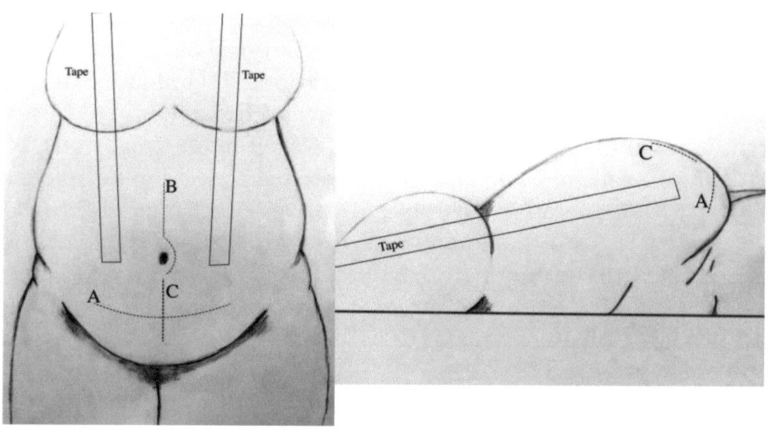

Figure 1.
Surgical skin incision choices. A – Pfannensteil, B – Supraumbilical, and C – Infraumbilical. The Pannus is elevated using tape bilaterally on the upper abdomen with gentle cephalad traction and anchored to the operating table. Care must be taken when choosing a lower abdominal incision (A or B) to avoid transecting the pannus.

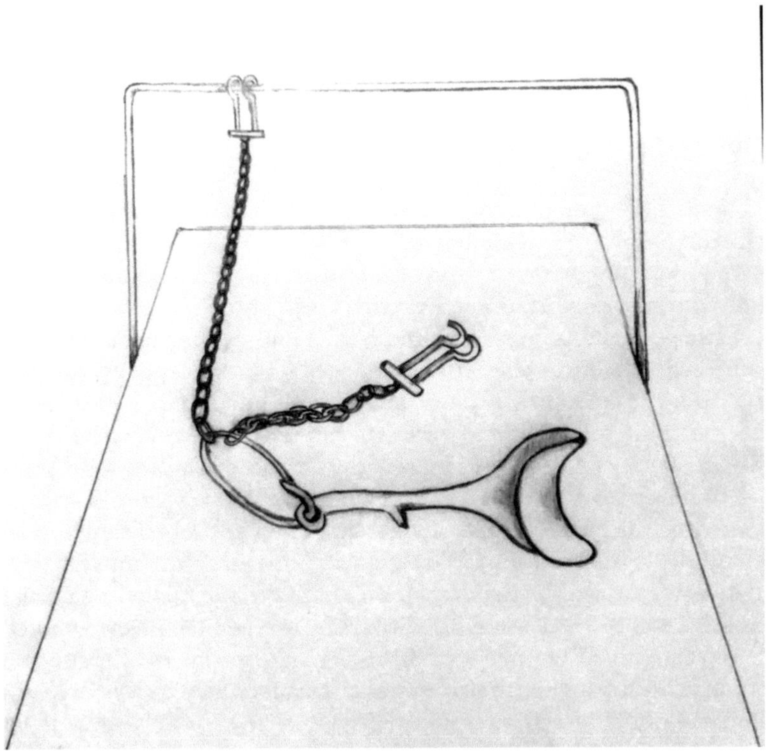

Figure 2.
Hook and doyen apparatus to retract pannus. The doyen retractor is attached with chains and hooks to a lateral bar on the operating table. The doyen retractor is placed under the pannus to elevate it out of the surgeon's way.

adjustable chain to attach a retractor placed under the pannus to a railing across the upper end of the operating table. Care must be used as the pannus is displaced on the maternal abdomen and may lead to hypotension and respiratory difficulties, especially if the patient is under regional anesthesia [64].

Longer operative time leads to increased chance of maternal complications including increased blood loss, transfusion, prolonged hospitalization and wound infection [32]. Unfortunately, the very nature of performing a cesarean section in the obese patient necessitates a longer surgery. Surgical techniques associated with shorter operative time may reduce complications. Techniques that favor blunt instead of sharp dissection reduce operative time, such as a modified Misgav-Ladach technique (limited sharp dissection in favor of blunt expansion), blunt expansion of the uterine incision, and finger-assisted stretching technique, or FAST [65–67]. Standardized operative technique also help reduce operative time [68]. Though not studied in obese women specifically, barbed sutures for uterine closure are also associated with shorter operative times [69].

Evidence suggests that closure of the subcutaneous tissue (if over 2–3 cm in depth) and avoidance of subcutaneous drains decrease the chance of wound complications in obese patients [70–72].

There is one known exception to the principle of reducing operative time to improve maternal outcomes. Subcuticular closure with suture reduces chances of wound complications, despite taking more time [73]. The choice of suture (4–0 vicryl or 4–0 monocryl) did not have an effect on wound complications in a randomized controlled trial with a large number (66%) of obese women [74].

6.4 Prevention of surgical site infections

Pre-operative antibiotic prophylaxis within 60 min and prior to skin incision has been associated with a significant reduction in surgical site infection in all women, regardless of their weight. However, the pharmacology of pre-operative antibiotics is altered in obese women. Higher doses of pre-operative antibiotics may be needed to prevent surgical site infection. Women with BMI $\geq$ 30 kg/m^2 may need 3 g of pre-operative cefazolin to achieve similar tissue concentrations of antibiotics as normal and overweight women [75–77]. The addition of a 48-h course of cephalexin and metronidazole in addition to the pre-operative cephalosporin IV prophylaxis has also been shown to reduce the chance of post-operative surgical site infection (within 30 days) in obese women [78].

The addition of azithromycin to standard antibiotic prophylaxis in women of all weight groups undergoing non-elective cesarean delivery has been proven to reduce wound infection [79]. Given the high chance of wound infection in obese patients, it may be reasonable to add azithromycin to standard antibiotic prophylaxis, even in women undergoing elective scheduled cesarean delivery [71]. In our institution, the addition of azithromycin has reduced surgical site infections in a longitudinal cohort quality improvement project (unpublished data).

Different types of skin incisions have not been definitively shown to reduce wound complications. Small studies have shown similar chance of wound complications in obese women with Pfannenstiel and vertical incisions, which is surprising given the moist and microbe rich environment that exists in the skin folds of the pannus [80]. A meta-analysis initially suggested vertical skin incisions may reduce chance of wound infection, but this article was subsequently redacted due to a miscalculation that favored Pfannenstiel for reducing risk of infection [81]. Evidence now suggests no clinical difference in outcomes of women with BMI $\geq$ 40 kg/m^2 who have either Pfannenstiel or vertical skin incisions [61].

Self-retaining retractors, unfortunately, have also not been found to reduce surgical site infection [30, 82].

As mentioned in Section 6.3, subcuticular closure with suture reduces chances of wound complications in obese women [73]. Skin closure with staples is associated with a higher chance of wound complication (infection, separation) in obese women within 6 weeks of delivery [83]. However, this effect did not persist in women with class III obesity (BMI $\geq$ 40 kg/m^2 [84]. The use of staples may be considered in super-obese women.

Many surgeons place prophylactic JP drains in the subcutaneous tissue of obese patients undergoing cesarean delivery, with the thought wound seromas and infection may be prevented. On a large multicenter randomized trial, obese women with subcutaneous drains had similar rates of wound complications as those with subcutaneous fat closure only [85]. However, more recent studies suggest that the subcutaneous tissue should be closed if more than 2–3 cm deep, and subcutaneous drains should be avoided to prevent surgical site infections [70–72].

Prophylactic administration of negative pressure wound therapy (Wound V.A.C.®, Prevena™) in obese patients with a BMI $\geq$ 40 kg/m^2 is associated with a reduction in surgical site infections [86]. Super-obese women may benefit from prophylactic application of negative pressure wound dressings, but a systematic review and meta-analysis suggests this strategy is not beneficial when cut offs for application are dropped to women with a BMI $\geq$ 30 kg/m^2 [87].

Despite implementation of known evidence based measures to prevent surgical site infection (prophylactic antibiotics within 60 min prior to skin incision, chlorhexidine –alcohol for skin antisepsis with 3 min of drying time before incision,

Weight (lb)	Dose (mg)*
200–240	50
241-290	60
291–330	70
331–370	80
371–400	90
>400	100

**Administered every 12 h. Adapted from Overcash et al. [95].*

Table 2.
Weight based enoxaparin dosing.

closure of subcutaneous tissue if ≥2 cm depth, and subcuticular skin closure with suture), surgical site infection remains high in obese women [88].

6.5 Prevention of venous thromboembolic events

Pneumatic compression devices, heparin, and low molecular weight heparin (LMWH) have all been suggested as strategies to reduce VTE in obese women undergoing cesarean delivery. Recommendations from major societies on the strategies for prevention of venous thromboembolism in obese women undergoing cesarean delivery are in conflict [89]. The American College of Obstetricians and Gynecologists (ACOG), the American College of Chest Physicians (ACCP), and the Royal College of Obstetricians and Gynecologists (RCOG) all differ slightly in their published recommendations. ACOG suggests all women undergoing cesarean delivery should use post-partum pneumatic compression devices, but gives no additional specific recommendations regarding obesity [90, 91]. The ACCP suggests obesity is a minor risk factor for VTE, and does not recommend post-partum pharmacoprophylaxis unless two minor risk factors are present [92]. In contrast, the RCOG suggests pharmacoprophylaxis should be administered to women with a BMI > 40 kg/m^2 who undergo a cesarean in labor.

Given their higher chance of post-operative VTE, it seems prudent to use at minimum pneumatic compression devices for VTE prophylaxis in obese women undergoing cesarean delivery, and has been found to be cost effective [93]. It seems reasonable to consider VTE pharmacoprophylaxis in women with BMI > 40 kg/m^2, though there is lack of evidence to strongly support this strategy [94]. It is equally important to consider that standard prophylactic doses may not be sufficient to achieve adequate concentrations due to the pharmacokinetics of LMWH in obese persons. Weight-based dosing of enoxaparin (0.5 mg/kg q 12 h) for prevention of thromboembolism is more effective than BMI-stratified dosing (BMI 40–59.9 received 40 mg enoxaparin q 12 h, BMI 60 received 60 mg q 12 h) in achieving adequate anti-Xa concentrations [95–97]. **Table 2** shows a weight-based enoxaparin dosing strategy for obese women.

7. Conclusion

Cesarean delivery occurs more often in obese women, and increases both maternal and neonatal morbidity. Adequate planning and preparation is required to perform a safe cesarean delivery in obese women, particularly in super-obese patients. Optimal, evidence-based practice includes:

- Adequate physical plant preparation with attention to sufficient equipment, policy, and staff training;
- Initiation of informed consent process during prenatal care visits or at time of admission, well in advance of operation;
- Anesthetic consideration and preparation for increased puncture time, number of punctures, high blocks, and difficult/high risk intubation;
- Selection of skin incision and attention to surgical techniques;
- Application of strategies to reduce post-operative wound complications; and
- Consideration of risk for and techniques to reduce risk for venous thromboembolism.

Despite adequate preparation and attention to prophylaxis against known adverse surgical outcomes, the obese patient will have elevated risk above her normal weight counterpart. Prevention of obesity, and adequate weight loss prior to conception is ultimately the best protection against complications at the time of cesarean delivery in the obese patient.

Acknowledgements

The authors acknowledge the artistry of Karen Skaret's illustrations included in this Chapter.

Conflict of interest

The authors have no conflicts of interest to report.

Author details

Kristina Roloff*, Suzanne Cao, Camille Okekpe, Inessa Dombrovsky and Guillermo Valenzuela
Department of Women's Health Arrowhead Regional Medical Center, Colton, CA, USA

*Address all correspondence to: kristyroloff@gmail.com

References

[1] Grasch J, Thompson J, Newton J, Zhai A, Osmundson S. Trial of labor compared with cesarean delivery in superobese women. Obstetrics and Gynecology. 2017;**130**(5):994-1000

[2] Wispelwey B, Sheiner E. Cesarean delivery in obese women: A comprehensive review. The Journal of Maternal-Fetal & Neonatal Medicine. 2013;**26**(6):547-551

[3] Borghesi Y, Labreuche J, Duhamel A, Pigeyre M, Deruelle P. Risk of cesarean delivery among pregnant women with class III obesity. International Journal of Gynaecology and Obstetrics. 2017;**136**(2):168-174

[4] Pettersen-Dahl A, Murzakanova G, Sandvik L, Laine K. Maternal body mass index as a predictor for delivery method. Acta Obstetricia et Gynecologica Scandinavica. 2018;**97**(2):212-218

[5] Kawakita T, Reddy U, Landy H, Iqbal S, Huang C, Grantz K. Indications for primary cesarean delivery relative to body mass index. American Journal of Obstetrics and Gynecology. 2016;**215**(4):515

[6] Gaudet L, Wen S, Walker M. The combined effect of maternal obesity and fetal macrosomia on pregnancy outcomes. Journal of Obstetrics and Gynaecology Canada. 2014;**36**(9):776-784

[7] Kominiarek M, Peaceman A. Gestational weight gain. American Journal of Obstetrics and Gynecology. 2017;**217**(6):642-651

[8] Zhao R, Xu L, Wu M, Huang S, Cao X. Maternal pre-pregnancy body mass index, gestational weight gain influence birth weight. Women and Birth. 2018;**31**(1):e20-e25

[9] Zhang C, Wu Y, Li S, Zhang D. Maternal prepregnancy obesity and the risk of shoulder dystocia: A meta-analysis. BJOG. 2018;**125**(4):407-413

[10] Kawatika T, Igbal S, Huang C, Reddy U. Nonmedically indicated induction in morbidly obese women is not associated with an increased risk of cesarean delivery. American Journal of Obstetrics and Gynecology. 2017;**217**(4):451

[11] Verdiales M, Pacheco C, Cohen W. The effect of maternal obesity on the course of labor. Journal of Perinatal Medicine. 2009;**37**(6):651-655

[12] Frolova A, Wang J, Conner S, Tuuli M, Macones G, Woolfolk C, et al. The obese patient has both an increased risk for needing an indicated cesarean delivery, and an increased risk for peri-operative complications. They are also at higher risk for failed trial of labor after cesarean delivery. American Journal of Perinatology. 2018;**35**(1):59-64

[13] Roloff K, Peng S, Sanchez-Ramos L, Valenzuela G. Cumulative oxytocin dose during induction of labor according to maternal body mass index. International Journal of Gynaecology and Obstetrics. 2015;**131**(1):54-58

[14] Carson N, Hernandez T, Hurt K. Parturition dysfunction in obesity: Time to target the pathobiology. Reproductive Biology and Endocrinology. 2015;**18**:13-135

[15] VanGompel E, Main E, Tancredi D, Melnikow J. Do provider birth attitudes influence cesarean delivery rate: A cross-sectional study. BMC Pregnancy and Childbirth. 2018;**18**:184

[16] Pulman K, Tohidi M, Pudell J, Davies G. Emergency caesarean section in obese Parturients: Is a 30-minute

decision-to-incision interval feasible? Journal of Obstetrics and Gynaecology Canada. 2015;**37**(11):988-994

[17] Girsen A, Osmundson S, Naqvi M, Garabedian M, Lyell D. Body mass index and operative times at cesarean delivery. Obstetrics and Gynecology. 2014;**124**(4):684-689

[18] Neumann K, Indorf I, Hartel C, Cirkel C, Rody A, Beyer D. C-section prevalence among obese mothers and neonatal Hypoglycemia: A cohort analysis of the Department of Gynecology and Obstetrics of the university of Lübeck. Geburtshilfe und Frauenheilkunde. 2017;**77**(5):487-494

[19] Metz T, Stoddard G, Henry E, Jackson M, Holmgren C, Esplin S. How do good candidates for trial of labor after cesarean (TOLAC) who undergo elective repeat cesarean differ from those who choose TOLAC? American Journal of Obstetrics and Gynecology. 2013;**208**(6):458.e1-458.e6

[20] Mourad M, Silverstein M, Bender S, Melka S, Klauser C, Gupta S, et al. The effect of maternal obesity on outcomes in patients undergoing tertiary or higher cesarean delivery. The Journal of Maternal-Fetal & Neonatal Medicine. 2015;**28**(9):989-993

[21] Roloff K, Gray A, Valenzuela G. Repeat cesarean delivery in the 39-week rule era: Outcomes at a community based hospital. Clinical and Experimental Obstetrics & Gynecology. 2017;**3**:391-395

[22] Smid M, Vladutiu C, Dotters-Katz S, Boggess K, Manuck T, Stamilio D. Maternal obesity and major intraoperative complications during cesarean delivery. American Journal of Obstetrics and Gynecology. 2017;**216**(6):614

[23] Smid M, Dotters-Katz S, Vaught A, Vladutiu C, Boggess K, Stamilio D. Maternal super obesity and risk for intensive care unit admission in the MFMU cesarean registry. Acta Obstetricia et Gynecologica Scandinavica. 2017;**96**(8):976-983

[24] Crane J, Murphy P, Burrage L, Hutchens D. Maternal and perinatal outcomes of extreme obesity in pregnancy. Journal of Obstetrics and Gynaecology Canada. 2013;**35**(7):606-611

[25] Smid M, Keaney M, Stamilio D. Extreme obesity and Postcesarean wound complications in the maternal-Fetal medicine unit Cesarean registry. American Journal of Perinatology. 2015;**32**(14):1336-1341

[26] Smid M, Dotters-Katz S, Silver R, Kuller J. Body mass index 50 kg/m2 and beyond: Perioperative Care of Pregnant Women with Superobesity Undergoing Cesarean Delivery. Obstetrical & Gynecological Survey. 2017;**72**(8):500-510

[27] Conner S, Verticchio J, Tuuli M, Odibo A, Macones G, Cahill A. Maternal obesity and risk of post-Cesarean wound complications. American Journal of Perinatology. 2014;**31**(4):299-304

[28] Tran T, Jamulitrat S, Chongsuvivatwong V, Geater A. Risk factors for postcesarean surgical site infection. Obstetrics and Gynecology. 2000;**95**(3):367-371

[29] Alanis M, Villers M, Law T, Steadman E, Robinson C. Complications of cesarean delivery in the massively obese parturient. American Journal of Obstetrics and Gynecology. 2010;**203**(3):271

[30] Yamasato K, Yoshino K, Chang A, Caughey A, Tsai P. Cesarean

delivery complications in women with morbid obesity. The Journal of Maternal-Fetal & Neonatal Medicine. 2016;**29**(23):3885-3888

[31] Väänänen A, Kainu J, Eriksson H, Lång M, Tekay A, et al. Does obesity complicate regional anesthesia and result in longer decision to delivery time for emergency cesarean section? Acta Anaesthesiologica Scandinavica. 2017;**61**(6):609-618

[32] Rottenstreich M, Sela H, Shen O, Michaelson-Cohen R, Samueloff A, Reichman O. Prolonged operative time of repeat cesarean is a risk marker for post-operative maternal complications. BMC Pregnancy and Childbirth. 2018;**18**(1):477

[33] Friedman A. Which risk factors for thromboembolism should guide obstetric prophylaxis? BJOG. 2019;**126**(5):589

[34] Simpson E, Lwrenson R, Nightingale A, Farmer R. Venous thromboembolism in pregnancy and the puerperium: Incidence and additional risk factors from a London perinatal database. BJOG : An International Journal of Obstetrics and Gynaecology. 2003;**108**(1):56-60

[35] Larsen T, Sorensen H, Gislum M, Johnsen S. Maternal smoking, obesity, and risk of venous thromboembolism during pregnancy and the puerperium: A population-based nested case-control study. Thrombosis Research. 2007;**120**(4):505-509

[36] Knight M. Antenatal pulmonary embolism: Risk factors, management and outcomes. BJOG : An International Journal of Obstetrics and Gynaecology. 2008;**115**(4):453-461

[37] Pomp E, Lenselink A, Rosendaal F, Doggen C. Pregnancy, the postpartum period and prothrombotic defects: Risk of venous thrombosis in the MEGA study. Journal of Thrombosis and Haemostasis. 2008;**6**(4):632-637

[38] Butwick A, Bentley J, Leonard S, Carmichael S, El-Sayed Y, Stephansson O, et al. Prepregnancy maternal body mass index and venous thromboembolism: A population-based cohort study. BJOG : An International Journal of Obstetrics and Gynaecology. 2019;**126**(5):581-588

[39] Jacobsen A, Skjeldestad F, Sandset P. Ante- and postnatal risk factors of venous thrombosis: A hospital-based case–control study. Journal of Thrombosis and Haemostasis. 2008;**6**:905-912

[40] Powell M, Morgan C, Cantu JSY, Biggio J, Tita A, Szychowski J, et al. Obesity and neonatal cord blood gas results at Cesarean: Effect of intraoperative blood pressure. American Journal of Perinatology. 2017;**34**(7):716-721

[41] Rimsza R, Perez W, Babbar S, O'Brien M, Vricella L. Time from neuraxial anesthesia placement to delivery is inversely proportional to umbilical arterial cord pH at scheduled cesarean delivery. American Journal of Obstetrics and Gynecology. 2019;**220**(4):389.e1-389.e9

[42] Smid M, Vladutiu C, Dotters-Katz S, Manuck T, Boggess K, Stamilio D. Maternal super obesity and neonatal morbidity after term Cesarean delivery. American Journal of Perinatology. 2016;**33**(12):1198-1204

[43] Conner S, Tuuli M, Longman R, Odibo A, Macones G, Cahill A. Impact of obesity on incision-to-delivery interval and neonatal outcomes at cesarean delivery. American Journal of Obstetrics and Gynecology. 2013;**209**(4):386

[44] Machado L. Cesarean section in morbidly obese Parturients: Practical implications and complications. North American Journal of Medical Sciences. 2012;**4**(1):13-18

[45] Hood D, Dewan D. Anesthetic and obstetric outcome in morbidly obese parturients. Anesthesiology. 1993;**79**(6):1210-1218

[46] Duvekott J. Pregnancy and obesity: Practical implications. European Clinics in Obstetrics and Gynaecology. 2005;**1**:74-88

[47] Lamon A, Habib A. Managing anesthesia for cesarean section in obese patients: Current perspectives. Local and Regional Anesthesia. 2016;**9**:45-57

[48] Simpson K. Perinatal patient safety: Extreme obesity as a patient safety risk during labor and birth. MCN. 2008;**33**(3):196

[49] Salmeen K, Brincat C. Time from consent to cesarean delivery during labor. American Journal of Obstetrics and Gynecology. 2013;**209**(3):212.e1-212.e6

[50] Raab E. The Paramters of informed consent. Transactions of the American Ophthalmological Society. 2004;**102**:225-232

[51] Kominiarek M, Gay F, Peacock N. Obesity in pregnancy: A qualitative approach to inform an intervention for patients and providers. Maternal and Child Health Journal. 2015;**19**(8):1698-1712

[52] An X, Zhao Y, Zhang Y, Yang Q, Wang Y, Cheng W, et al. Risk assessment of morbidly obese parturient in cesarean section delivery: A prospective, cohort, single-center study. Medicine. 2017;**96**(42):e8265

[53] Lamon A, Einhorn L, Cooter M, Habib A. The impact of body mass index on the risk of high spinal block in parturients undergoing cesarean delivery: A retrospective cohort study. Journal of Anesthesia. 2017;**31**(4):552-558

[54] Ngaka T, Coetzee J, Dyer R. The influence of body mass index on sensorimotor block and vasopressor requirement during spinal anesthesia for elective cesarean delivery. Anesthesia and Analgesia. 2016;**123**(6):1527-1534

[55] Urfalioğlu A, Bilal B, Öksüz G, Bakacak M, Boran Ö, Öksüz H. Comparison of the landmark and ultrasound methods in cesarean sections performed under spinal anesthesia on obese pregnants. The Journal of Maternal-Fetal & Neonatal Medicine. 2017;**30**(9):1051-1056

[56] Sahin T, Balaban O, Sahin L, Solak M, Toker K. A randomized controlled trial of preinsertion ultrasound guidance for spinal anaesthesia in pregnancy: Outcomes among obese and lean parturients: Ultrasound for spinal anesthesia in pregnancy. Journal of Anesthesia. 2014;**25**(3):413-419

[57] Roofhooft E. Anesthesia for the morbidly obese parturient. Current Opinion in Anaesthesiology. 2009;**22**:341-346

[58] Mace H, Paech MMN. Obesity and obstetric anaesthesia. Anaesthesia and Intensive Care. 2011;**39**(4):559-570

[59] Brocato B, Thorpe E, Gomez L, Wan J, Mari G. The effect of cesarean delivery skin incision approach in morbidly obese women on the rate of classical hysterotomy. Journal of Pregnancy. 2013;**2013**:1-3

[60] Sutton A, Sanders LS, Jauk V, Edwards R. Abdominal incision selection for Cesarean delivery

of women with class III obesity. American Journal of Perinatology. 2016;**33**(6):547-551

[61] Marrs C, Blackwell S, Hester A, Olson G, Saade G, Faro J, et al. Pfannenstiel versus vertical skin incision for Cesarean delivery in women with class III obesity: A randomized trial. American Journal of Perinatology. 2019;**36**(1):97-104

[62] Smid M, Smiley S, Schulkin J, Stamilio D, Edwards R, Stuebe A. The problem of the Pannus: Physician preference survey and a review of the literature on Cesarean skin incision in morbidly obese women. American Journal of Perinatology. 2016;**33**(5):463-472

[63] Smid M, Edwards R, Biggio J, Dorman K, Leduke R, Lesher L, et al. Class III obese Women's preferences and concerns for Cesarean skin incision: A Multicenter survey. American Journal of Perinatology. 2017;**34**(3):289-294

[64] Viegas C, Viegas O. Preventing a surgical complication during Cesarean delivery in a morbidly obese patient: A simple apparatus to retract the abdominal Panniculus. MedGenMed. 2006;**8**(1):52

[65] Saad A, Rahman M, Costantine M, Saade G. Blunt versus sharp uterine incision expansion during low transverse cesarean delivery: A metaanalysis. American Journal of Obstetrics and Gynecology. 2014;**211**(6):684

[66] Hudić I, Bujold E, Fatušić Z, Skokić F, Latifagić A, Kapidžić M, et al. The Misgav-Ladach method of cesarean section: A step forward in operative technique in obstetrics. Archives of Gynecology and Obstetrics. 2012;**286**(5):1141-1146

[67] Song S, Oh M, Kim T, Hur J, Saw H, Park Y. Finger-assisted stretching technique for cesarean section. International Journal of Gynaecology and Obstetrics. 2006;**92**(3):212-216

[68] Pallister M, Ballas J, Kohn J, Eppes C, Belfort M, Davidson C. Standardized approach to Cesarean surgical technique and its effect on operative time and surgical morbidity. American Journal of Perinatology. 2019;**36**(3):277-284

[69] Zayed M, Fouda U, Elsetohy K, Zayed S, Hashem A, Youssef M. Barbed sutures versus conventional sutures for uterine closure at cesarean section; a randomized controlled trial. The Journal of Maternal-Fetal & Neonatal Medicine. 2017;**29**:1-8

[70] Ayres-de-Campos D. Obesity and the challenges of caesarean delivery: Prevention and management of wound complications. Best Practice & Research. Clinical Obstetrics & Gynaecology. 2015;**29**(3):406-414

[71] Kawakita T, Landy H. Surgical site infections after cesarean delivery: Epidemiology, prevention and treatment. Maternal Health, Neonatology and Perinatology. 2017;**3**:12

[72] Ramsey P, White A, Guinn D, Lu G, Ramin S, Davies J, et al. Subcutaneous tissue reapproximation, alone or in combination with drain, in obese women undergoing cesarean delivery. Obstetrics and Gynecology. 2005;**105** (5 pt 1):967-973

[73] Mackeen A, Khalifeh A, Fleisher J, Vogell A, Han C, Sendecki J, et al. Suture compared with staple skin closure after cesarean delivery: A randomized controlled trial. Obstetrics and Gynecology. 2014;**123**(6):1169-1175

[74] Tuuli M, Stout M, Martin S, Rampersad R, Cahill A, Macones G. Comparison of suture materials for subcuticular skin closure at cesarean delivery. American Journal of Obstetrics

and Gynecology. 2016;**215**(4):490.e1-490.e5

[75] Swank M, Wing D, Nicolau D, McNulty J. Increased 3-gram cefazolin dosing for cesarean delivery prophylaxis in obese women. American Journal of Obstetrics and Gynecology. 2015;**213**(3):415

[76] Young O, Shaik I, Twedt R, Binstock A, Althouse A, Venkataramanan R, et al. Pharmacokinetics of cefazolin prophylaxis in obese gravidae at time of cesarean delivery. American Journal of Obstetrics and Gynecology. 2015;**213**(4):541

[77] Kram J, Greer D, Cabrera O, Burlage R, Forgie M, Siddiqui D. Does current cefazolin dosing achieve adequate tissue and blood concentrations in obese women undergoing cesarean section? European Journal of Obstetrics, Gynecology, and Reproductive Biology. 2017;**210**:334-341

[78] Valent A, DeArmond C, Houston J, Reddy S, Masters H, Gold A, et al. Effect of post-Cesarean delivery Oral cephalexin and metronidazole on surgical site infection among obese women: A randomized clinical trial. Journal of the American Medical Association. 2017;**318**(11):1026-1034

[79] Tita A, Szychowski J, Boggess K, Saade G, Longo S, Clark E, et al. Adjunctive azithromycin prophylaxis for Cesarean delivery. The New England Journal of Medicine. 2016;**375**(13):1231-1341

[80] McLean M, Hines R, Polinkovsky M, Stuebe A, Thorp J, Strauss R. Ype of skin incision and wound complications in the obese parturient. American Journal of Perinatology. 2012;**29**(4):301-306

[81] Marrs C, Moussa H, Sibai B, Blackwell S. REMOVED: The relationship between primary cesarean delivery skin incision type and wound complications in women with morbid obesity. American Journal of Obstetrics and Gynecology. 2014;**210**(4):319

[82] Scolari Childress K, Gavard J, Ward D, Berger K, Gross G. A barrier retractor to reduce surgical site infections and wound disruptions in obese patients undergoing cesarean delivery: A randomized controlled trial. American Journal of Obstetrics and Gynecology. 2016;**214**(2):285

[83] Zaki M, Truong M, Pyra M, Kominiarek M, Irwin T. Wound complications in obese women after cesarean: A comparison of staples versus subcuticular suture. Journal of Perinatology. 2016;**36**(10):819-822

[84] Zaki M, Wing D, McNulty J. Comparison of staples vs subcuticular suture in class III obese women undergoing cesarean: A randomized controlled trial. American Journal of Obstetrics and Gynecology. 2018;**218**(4):451

[85] Ramsey P, White A, Guinn D, Lu G, Ramin S, Davies J, et al. Subcutaneous tissue reapproximation, alone or in combination with drain, in obese women undergoing cesarean delivery. Obstetrics and Gynecology. 2005;**105**(5 Pt 1):967-973

[86] Looby M, Vogel R, Bangdiwala A, Hyer B, Das K. Prophylactic negative pressure wound therapy in obese patients following Cesarean delivery. Surgical Innovation. 2018;**25**(1):43-49

[87] Smid M, Dotters-Katz S, Grace M, Wright S, Villers M, Hardy-Fairbanks A, et al. Prophylactic negative pressure wound therapy for obese women after Cesarean delivery: A systematic review and meta-analysis. Obstetrics and Gynecology. 2017;**130**(5):969-978

[88] Temming L, Raghuraman N, Carter E, Stout M, Rampersad R, Macones G, et al. Impact of evidence-based

interventions on wound complications after cesarean delivery. American Journal of Obstetrics and Gynecology. 2017;**217**(4):449

[89] Friedman A, Ananth C. Obstetrical venous thromboembolism: Epidemiology and strategies for prophylaxis. Seminars in Perinatology. 2016;**40**(2):81-86

[90] James A. Committee on practice bulletins-obstetrics. Practice bulletin No. 138: Inherited Thrombophilias in pregnancy. Obstetrics and Gynecology. 2013;**122**(3):706-716

[91] American College of Obstetricians and Gynecologisits Women's Health Care Physicians. ACOG practice bulletin No. 138: Inherited Thrombophilias in pregnancy. Obstetrics and Gynecology. 2013;**122**:706-717

[92] Bates S, Greer I, Middeldorp S, Veenstra D, Prabulos A, Vandvik P. VTE, thrombophilia, antithrombotic therapy, and pregnancy. Chest. 2012;**141**(2):619-763

[93] Casele H, Grobman W. Cost-effectiveness of thromboprophylaxis with intermittent pneumatic compression at cesarean delivery. Obstetrics and Gynecology. 2006;**108** (3 pt 1):535-540

[94] Catalano P, Shankar K. Obesity and pregnancy: Mechanisms of short term and long term adverse consequences for mother and child. BMJ. 2017;**356**:j1

[95] Overcash R, Somers A, LaCoursier D. Enoxaparin dosing after cesarean delivery in morbidly obese women. Obstetrics and Gynecology. 2015;**125**(6):1371-1376

[96] Conner S, Verticchio J, Methodius G, Odibo A, Macones G, Cahill A. Maternal obesity and risk of post-cesarean wound complications. American Journal of Perinatology. 2014;**31**(4):299-304

[97] Subramaniam A, Jauk V, Goss A, Alvarez M, Reese C, Edwards R. Mode of delivery in women with class III obesity: Planned cesarean compared with induction of labor. American Journal of Obstetrics and Gynecology. 2014;**11**(6):700

Chapter 6

Caesarean Section in Low-, Middle- and High-Income Countries

Josaphat Byamugisha and Moses Adroma

Abstract

Caesarean section (CS) refers to delivery of a foetus through surgical incisions made through abdominal and uterine walls. It's a life-saving procedure when complications arise during pregnancy. It may be an emergency or a planned procedure. Although desirable, CS may be medically unnecessary. CS is a major procedure associated with immediate and long-term maternal and perinatal risks and may have implications for future pregnancies. Since 1985, international healthcare community considers ideal rate for CS to be 10–15%. However, in the last decade, there has been concern about the rising rates of CS from as low as 2% in Africa to as high as 50–60% in Dominican Republic and Latin America. To this effect, there have been attempts to regulate the rates, and the Ten Group Classification System under the Robson criteria is such an attempt. CS rates are on the increase due to varying reasons ranging from patient, institutional, care provider and societal factors. There have been modifications in the CS technique and the drugs used postoperatively from Pitocin to addition of Misoprostol. Need has developed from Reproductive Health Specialists to review indications, rates and terminologies used and evaluate practices in low-, middle- and high-income countries regarding CS.

Keywords: caesarean section, rates, LMICs

1. Definition

Caesarean delivery commonly referred to as caesarean section and occasionally caesarean birth is defined as the delivery of a foetus(es) through surgical incisions made through the anterior abdominal wall (technically referred to as laparotomy) and the anterior uterine wall (technically denoted to as hysterotomy) [1, 2]. This definition considers only the intrauterine location of the foetus and not whether the foetus is delivered alive or dead [3]. Since the words "caesarean" and "section" are both derived from verbs that mean to cut, some authors [1] urge that the phrase "caesarean section" is a tautology. Consequently, the terms "caesarean delivery" and "caesarean birth" are preferable.

Although infrequent, there are reports of foetal survival from advanced abdominal pregnancies resulting into live birth [4]. The procedure for delivery of such foetus(es) is not caesarean section but rather laparotomy. It is technically challenging to assign the type of procedure carried when simultaneous abdominal and intrauterine pregnancy is encountered [5]. Considering the definitions above, it would be urged that the procedure is caesarean section for the intrauterine foetus and laparotomy for the abdominal pregnancy. However, laparotomy alone would suffice. Confusion also arises among medical students when a foetus before the age of viability has to be delivered through abdominal surgery. Most obstetricians and gynaecologists refer to this procedure as hysterotomy rather than caesarean section.

2. Origin of word caesarean section and additional background of caesarean section

Caesarean section has been recorded in history since ancient times in both Western and non-Western literature. Although the first use of the term in obstetrics was from the seventeenth century, its early history is obscured by mythology [6]. Many historians believe that the origin of the term caesarean section rather than caesarean is from the birth of Gaius Julius Caesar [3]. This belief has been challenged by many.

To start with, Gaius Julius Caesar certainly was not the first person born via caesarean section. The procedure, or something close to it, is mentioned in the history and legend of various civilizations from Europe to the Far East well before his birth. He was not even the first Roman born that way. By the time Gaius Julius Caesar entered the world, Romans were already performing caesarean sections, and the Roman law reserved the operation for women who died in childbirth (so that the woman and her baby could be buried separately) and as a last resort for living mothers in order to save the baby's life during deliveries with complications. In ancient times, it was performed only when the woman was dead or dying as an attempt to rescue the foetus. This annuls further the origin of the term from Gaius Julius Caesar because his mother Aurelia Cotta is known to have lived long enough to see her son reach adulthood and serve him as a political advisor. Some sources even suggest she outlived him and he had two sisters, one of whom at least was younger than him [2].

Another possible source for the term is the Latin verb *caedare*, meaning to cut, or the term for the children who were born by postmortem caesarean sections, who were called *caesones*. The Roman law, Lex Regis, which dates from 600 BC, required that infants be delivered abdominally after maternal death to facilitate separate burial. This has also been proposed as the origin of the term. The specific law in question was called the Lex Cesare [7].

Historical records claim that the earliest authenticated report of a child who survived caesarean birth is a document describing the birth of Gorgias in Sicily in approximately 508 BC [7]. During this time period, the caesarean operation remained crude at best. The abdominal incision was made lateral to the rectus muscles, and the uterus was incised at whichever portion was accessible through the laparotomy incision. The uterine musculature was not reapproximated, and the patient had to be physically restrained during the procedure because of unavailability of anaesthesia [2]. As operative techniques improved, caesarean section became safer and could be used at an earlier stage in difficult labours. Further modifications emerged including emptying the bladder and rectum preoperatively with catheters and enemas, respectively, to decrease the volume of these organs in the operative field, thereby reducing the risk of injury during the surgical procedure [2].

3. Indications for caesarean section

Caesarean delivery is performed when the clinician and patient feel that abdominal delivery is likely to provide a better maternal and/or foetal outcome than vaginal delivery. Indications for caesarean delivery vary depending on the clinical situation, resources available for patient care, and individual physician management techniques. There are no definitive algorithms available to the practicing obstetrician to direct when an abdominal delivery will benefit the mother and/or the foetus in every clinical situation. The decision to perform an abdominal delivery therefore remains a joint judgement between the physician and patient after carefully weighing the pros and cons of a caesarean delivery versus continued labour and/or operative or spontaneous vaginal delivery [3]. Some authors have suggested that the term "elective caesarean delivery" should probably be eliminated because a caesarean delivery is either "medically/obstetrically indicated" or "on maternal request" and never truly "elective" [8].

The decision to perform an indicated caesarean delivery may be made antepartum (scheduled caesarean delivery) or as a result of concerns identified after labour has begun ("unscheduled caesarean delivery" or "unplanned caesarean delivery"). The terms "scheduled caesarean delivery" and "planned caesarean delivery" are used when the decision to perform a caesarean delivery does not occur as a consequence of a complication of labour but is planned antepartum such as in the case of repeat caesarean delivery, foetal malpresentation or placenta praevia. This therefore means that indications for caesarean delivery can be divided into indications that are of benefit to the mother (maternal indications), the foetus (foetal indications) or both (circumstances in which both foetal and maternal indications exist).

The indications can be further divided into absolute and relative indication in each of the maternal and foetal categories. Indications for caesarean delivery for maternal benefit include any situation in which it is inadvisable to continue to strive for a vaginal delivery out of concern for maternal outcome. In these situations, the woman undergoes a major abdominal operation for indications that are likely to decrease her risk for morbidity and/or mortality. In contrast, when a caesarean section is performed for foetal indications, the mother is undergoing major abdominal surgery when there is no immediate benefit to her but there is potential benefit to the neonate. In these situations, foetal health would be compromised if further efforts toward vaginal delivery were pursued [3].

3.1 Maternal indications

1. Previous hysterotomy (usually related to caesarean delivery, but also related to myomectomy or other uterine surgery). In the case of prior caesarean delivery, two prior caesarean deliveries are an absolute indication. However, women with one prior caesarean delivery can be offered trial of labour if there is no additional risk to vaginal delivery [1, 3, 8, 9].

2. Obstructive lesions in the lower genital tract including malignancies, condyloma acuminata, severely displaced pelvic fracture and leiomyomas of the lower uterine segment that interfere with the engagement of the foetal head.

3. Maternal infection (e.g. herpes simplex virus or human immunodeficiency virus (HIV)).

4. Prior classical hysterotomy.

5. Unknown uterine scar type.

6. Uterine incision dehiscence.

7. Prior full thickness myomectomy.

8. Genital tract obstructive mass.
9. Invasive cervical cancer.
10. Prior trachelectomy.
11. Permanent cerclage.
12. Prior pelvic reconstructive surgery.
13. Prior significant perineal trauma.
14. Pelvic deformity.
15. Cardiac or pulmonary disease.
16. Cerebral aneurysm or arteriovenous malformations.
17. Pathology requiring concurrent intra-abdominal surgery.
18. Perimortem caesarean delivery.

3.2 Foetal indications

1. Non-reassuring foetal status [1].
2. Foetal malpresentation.
3. Foetal bleeding diathesis.
4. Funic presentation or cord prolapse [3].
5. Macrosomia.
6. Abnormal lies or nonvertex presentations [8].
7. Multiple pregnancies: the first twin in a nonvertex presentation or higher-order multiples (triplets or greater).
8. Some congenital anomalies.
9. Foetal compromise [9].
10. Maternal infection: primary genital herpes and HIV.
11. Abnormal umbilical cord Doppler study.
12. Thrombocytopenia.
13. Prior neonatal birth trauma.
14. Caesarean delivery may be performed but is not routinely indicated for foetal issues, such as extremely or very low birth weight (<1000 g and ≤ 1500 g, respectively) [10].

15. Some individuals also consider caesarean delivery for certain congenital anomalies (e.g. open neural tube defects, some skeletal dysplasia and gastroschisis with herniated liver) [11, 12].

3.3 Both maternal and foetal indications

1. Failure to progress during labour [1].

2. Abnormal placentation (e.g. placenta praevia, vasa praevia, placenta accreta) [3].

3. Obstructed labour.

4. Cephalopelvic disproportion.

5. Failed operative vaginal delivery [8].

6. Abruption placenta with a live baby [9].

There are no absolute contraindications to caesarean delivery. In contrast to other types of surgery, the risks and benefits of the procedure need to be considered as they apply to two patients. However, many pregnant women have a low tolerance for accepting any foetal risk from vaginal birth, irrespective of the maternal risks associated with operative intervention [13].

4. Classification of caesarean section

Traditionally, caesarean section has been classified as emergency or elective. However, with advanced practice in obstetrics and more complicated deliveries encountered, this definition has become too simplistic, and more detailed categories are needed. Some authors have also suggested that the term "elective caesarean delivery" should probably be eliminated because a caesarean delivery is either "medically/obstetrically indicated" or "on maternal request" and never truly "elective" [8]. Such authors advocate for terms as *scheduled or planned* caesarean delivery in which the decision to perform an indicated caesarean delivery may be made antepartum and *unscheduled or unplanned* caesarean section where decision to perform an indicated caesarean delivery is made as a result of concerns identified after labour has begun. The decision to perform an unscheduled caesarean section may also arise even when labour has not occurred such as in abruption placentae with a live baby and no labour pains or absent foetal movement with abnormal umbilical artery Doppler studies not in labour.

Also distinguishing between prelabour caesarean section (which may be scheduled/elective or emergency/unscheduled) and intrapartum caesarean delivery (which is, by default, emergency) is preferable [14].

Lucas and colleagues [15] developed the classification of caesarean delivery based on urgency approved by the Royal College of Obstetricians and Gynaecologists (RCOG) and the Royal College of Anaesthetists in the UK after it was developed further into the most consistent method recommended by National Confidential Enquiry into Perioperative Deaths [16].

The initial classification by Lucas et al. [15] was a four-grade classification system including:

Classification	Indication
Grade 1: emergency caesarean section	Immediate threat to the life of the woman or the foetus, i.e. placental abruption (antepartum) or uterine rupture (intrapartum)
Grade 2: urgent caesarean section	No immediate risk to the life of the woman or baby, but delivery should be achieved as soon as possible, e.g. three previous caesarean sections, membranes are ruptured with meconium-stained liquor (antepartum) or non-reassuring cardiotocograph and foetal blood sampling are not possible or contraindicated
Grade 3: nonscheduled caesarean section	Delivery is needed but can fit in with delivery suite workload and allow for fasting/steroid administration and some degree of planning, e.g. preterm intrauterine growth restriction, preeclampsia, etc.
Grade 4: scheduled, also referred to as elective caesarean section	No urgency whatsoever and procedure planned to suit the mother, staff, delivery suite, etc. and carried out at 39 weeks' gestation during the working day (i.e. not out of hours)

Reproduced from The Global Library of Women's Medicine.

Table 1.
Classification of caesarean section.

1. Immediate threat to life of woman or foetus

2. Maternal or foetal compromise which is not immediately life-threatening

3. Needing early delivery but no maternal or foetal compromise

4. At a time to suit the patient and maternity team

Based on this the following classification of caesarean delivery was proposed (**Table 1**) [3].

5. Techniques for caesarean section

Caesarean operation has undergone a number of technical changes as the procedure has evolved. Many different practitioners extol the benefits of various techniques of skin incision, uterine incision, uterine closure, and many other technical aspects of the operation. However, there are relatively few randomised trials to support many of the commonly used practices at caesarean section. As such there is no standard technique for caesarean delivery although there are a few evidence-based recommendations for the surgical technique.

5.1 Abdominal opening

Abdominal opening is accomplished through either transverse (Pfannenstiel and Joel-Cohen) or vertical skin incisions, each of which has advantages and disadvantages. Incision of about 12–15 cm is usually adequate for access [3, 14]. Historically, a vertical midline skin incision was implemented; however, this scar is cosmetically less acceptable and is associated with higher incidence of postoperative wound discomfort, dehiscence, infection, and hernia formation [3]. It may still be necessary if access is required to the upper uterus or to other abdominal organs. At present, the most frequently used type of skin incision is the Pfannenstiel incision since it is associated with less postoperative pain, greater wound strength and better cosmetic results than the vertical midline incision [17]. The use of scalpel is preferred although there are no randomised trials comparing scalpel to electrocautery which can also be used during caesarean delivery.

Opening the subcutaneous tissue layer is achieved bluntly preferred to sharp dissection as blunt dissection has been associated with shorter operative times and less chance of injury to vessels [18]. However, there are no randomised trials comparing techniques for incision and dissection of the subcutaneous tissues at caesarean delivery.

There are no randomised trials comparing different techniques of opening the fascia. A small transverse incision is usually made medially with the scalpel and then extended laterally with scissors. Alternatively, the fascial incision can be extended bluntly by inserting the fingers of each hand under the fascia and then pulling in a cephalad-caudad direction [17, 18].

Rectus muscles are separated bluntly in most cases. Avoiding transection of muscles preserves muscle strength. Dissection of the rectus fascia from the rectus sheath and muscles is unnecessary [19] but has not been studied separately in a randomised trial.

Opening the peritoneum can be achieved using the fingers bluntly to minimise the risk of inadvertent injury to the bowel, bladder or other organs that may be adherent to the underlying surface [18, 19]. However blunt versus sharp entry into the peritoneum has not been compared in a randomised trial.

5.2 Hysterotomy/opening the uterus

Opening of the bladder flap may or may not be performed. Some surgeons choose to open the bladder flap if difficult delivery is anticipated such as when the foetal head is deep in the pelvis or when the bladder is attached well above the lower uterine segment after a previous caesarean delivery. In these cases, creation of the bladder flap may help to keep the bladder dome out of the surgical field if the uterine incision extends.

The uterine incision may be transverse or vertical. The type of incision depends upon several factors, including the position and size of the foetus, location of the placenta, presence of leiomyomas and development of the lower uterine segment. The principal consideration is that the incision must be large enough to allow atraumatic delivery of the foetus. Transverse incision along the lower uterine segment is recommended. Compared with vertical incisions, advantages of the transverse incision include less blood loss, less need for bladder dissection, easier approximation and a lower risk of rupture in subsequent pregnancies [19]. Low vertical and classical incisions may also be performed in certain circumstances. Low vertical incision is performed in the lower uterine segment and appears to be as strong as the low transverse incision [20]. The major disadvantage of the low vertical incision is the possibility of extension cephalad into the uterine fundus or caudally into the bladder, cervix or vagina. It is also difficult to determine that the low vertical incision is truly low, as the separation between lower and upper uterine segments is not easily identifiable clinically. Classical incision is rarely performed at or near term because in subsequent pregnancies it is associated with a higher frequency of uterine dehiscence/rupture than low vertical and low transverse incisions. The generally accepted indications for considering a vertical uterine incision are:

- Poorly developed lower uterine segment in a setting in which more than normal intrauterine manipulation is anticipated (e.g. extremely preterm breech presentation, back down transverse lie)

- Lower uterine segment pathology that precludes a transverse incision (e.g. large leiomyoma, anterior placenta praevia or accreta)

- Densely adherent bladder

- Postmortem delivery

5.3 Delivery of the baby and placenta

Extraction of the foetus at caesarean delivery is usually uncomplicated but may be made more difficult by extreme prematurity, a deeply impacted or floating foetal head or an abnormal lie. However, careful attention to the duration of prolonged uterine incision to delivery time is important especially in a foetus with a non-reassuring foetal heart rate assessment prior to the onset of surgery.

Cord clamping. Delayed, rather than immediate, cord clamping results in greater neonatal haemoglobin levels and appears to be beneficial for preterm, and some term, infants. However, in asphyxiated baby, the cord should be quickly clamped and cut.

Delivery of the placenta is best achieved with controlled cord traction and aided by oxytocin administration instead of manual delivery which is associated with postoperative endometritis and greater blood loss. To ensure that all of the placenta has been removed, the uterus is usually explored with one hand holding a sponge to remove any remaining membranes or placental tissue, while the other hand is placed on the fundus to stabilise the uterus. These manipulations further stimulate uterine contraction.

5.4 Closure of the uterus

The uterus may or may not be exteriorized. No approach is superior to the other. Closing the uterus after caesarean section is best performed with a double-layer technique using continuous closure with delayed absorbable synthetic suture incorporating all of the muscle in order to avoid bleeding from the incision edges. Some obstetricians prefer locking the sutures instead of continuous [21]. Recently, Lambert's suture technique for the second layer is being promoted. The bladder peritoneum may or may not reperitonised.

5.5 Closure of the abdomen

The peritoneal layer may or may not be closed. Nonclosure might allow the enlarged uterus to adhere to the anterior abdominal wall or impede spontaneous closure of the peritoneum, while closure might cause a foreign body reaction to sutures and tissue damage [22]. A systematic review of peritoneal nonclosure and adhesion formation after caesarean delivery found some evidence that nonclosure was associated with greater adhesion formation than closure of the parietal layer or both visceral and parietal layers [23].

Rectus muscles are believed to reapproximate naturally, and suturing them together may cause unnecessary pain when the woman starts to move after surgery [17]. There is no randomised trial that has evaluated rectus muscle closure versus nonclosure.

Fascial closure is a critical aspect of incisional closure as this provides the majority of wound strength during healing. Care should be taken to avoid too much tension when closing the fascia since reapproximation, not strangulation, is the goal. The closure is best achieved with a simple running technique using no 1 or 2 delayed absorbable monofilament suture [22].

The subcutaneous adipose layer is closed with interrupted delayed absorbable sutures if the layer is ≥ 2 cm. Closure of the dead space seems to inhibit accumulation of serum and blood, which can lead to a wound seroma and subsequent wound breakdown [24]. The point of this layer is to support the skin layer, so Scarpa's fascia should be deliberately included in it [14].

Reapproximation of the skin may be performed with staples or subcuticular suture. No approach is superior to the other [25] although stables are associated with a doubling of wound complications (infection and wound separation) [26]. Subcuticular stitches have been associated with less immediate postoperative pain and are more cosmetically appealing at 6 weeks than the stapling device [27]. For subcuticular suture, absorbable sutures such as Vicryl may be used.

6. Complications of caesarean section

Although a life-saving procedure for either the mother or the baby or both, caesarean section comes with a number of complications including but not limited to [28]:

1. Infections including endometritis and wound infections. Necrotizing fasciitis is rare but can occur after caesarean section.

2. Septic pelvic thrombophlebitis including ovarian vein thrombophlebitis and deep septic pelvic thrombophlebitis.

3. Haemorrhage. The mean blood loss at caesarean is approximately 1000 mL; however, estimates of blood loss are not very reliable.

4. Urinary tract and blood problems including ileus, urinary tract and bowel injuries.

5. Venous thrombosis and embolism whose risk is increased during the postoperative period. Early ambulation and thromboprophylaxis for high-risk mothers are recommended to decrease the risk of thromboembolism.

6. Disruption (or opening) of the caesarean laparotomy wound is common, especially in women with risk factors such as obesity, diabetes, history of wound disruption, vertical incision, etc.

7. Foetal and neonatal birth risks such as iatrogenic prematurity and birth trauma, transient tachypnea of the newborn, respiratory distress syndrome, etc.

8. Maternal mortality.

9. Abnormal placentation in subsequent pregnancy.

10. Subfertility. Women whose first birth is by caesarean are less likely to have a subsequent pregnancy than women whose first birth is a spontaneous vaginal delivery.

11. Scar complications including hysterotomy scar pregnancy, numbness and incisional endometriosis.

12. Uterine rupture in a subsequent pregnancy.

13. Abdominal adhesions that may predispose to bowel obstruction, strangulation, infertility and visceral injury during subsequent abdominal operations.

7. Caesarean section rates and why the increase over the decades

The international healthcare community has considered the ideal rate for caesarean sections to be between 10 and 15% [29] based on a 1985 WHO meeting in Brazil that stated that there is no justification for any region to have a rate higher than 10–15%. Since then caesarean sections have become increasingly common in both developed and developing countries for a variety of reasons [30].

When medically justified, caesarean section can effectively prevent maternal and perinatal mortality and morbidity. However, there is no evidence showing the benefits of caesarean delivery for women or infants who do not require the procedure. The proportion of caesarean sections at the population level is a measure of the level of access to and use of this intervention. It can serve as a guideline for policy-makers and governments in assessing progress in maternal and infant health and in monitoring emergency obstetric care and resource use.

Concerns on the rise in the numbers of caesarean section births and the potential negative consequences for maternal and infant health have been raised [31]. This concern is extended also to cost which is a major factor in improving equitable access to maternal and newborn care, as caesarean sections represent significant expense for overloaded and often weakened health system. However, determining the adequate caesarean section rate at the population level, i.e. the minimum rate for medically or obstetrically indicated caesarean section, while avoiding medically unnecessary operations is a challenging task.

In the United States, the caesarean delivery rate rose from 4.5% in 1970 to 32.9% in 2009. Following this peak, the rate has trended slightly downward, and it was 32.0% in 2015 [9]. In China the caesarean section rate was 42% in 2010 [31] despite the author claiming it had reduced. The rates can be even higher in private clinics. For example, in Brazil, 80–90% of births in private clinics are now caesarean sections, compared with about 30–40% of births in public hospitals [32]. Countries with high caesarean section rates include the Dominican Republic 56.4%, Brazil 55.6%, Egypt 51.8%, Turkey 50.4%, Iran 47.9% and China 47%.

See more at https://www.bellybelly.com.au/birth/highest-c-section-rates-by-country/.

At the other end of the spectrum, sub-Saharan Africa is still struggling to give mothers access to caesarean sections when required. Across this region, the caesarean section rate has changed very little since 2000, hovering right around 5%. This also varies from country to country and from private to public hospitals. In Africa only 7.3% of babies are born via this method. But it is a very mixed picture across the continent. Some countries have very high rates such as Egypt (51.8%) and Mauritius (47%), the highest in Africa. And despite a 2.9% overall increase across the continent from 1990, there has been a decline in some countries like Nigeria and Guinea which now stands at about 2%. Zimbabwe has maintained its caesarean section rates at 6%.

So what is driving the global rise of Caesarean sections? Some scholars claim it is likely three factors working together: financial, legal and technical with some people calling for hospitals to pay doctors equally for vaginal births in order to bring these rates down. However, the reasons for persistently significant caesarean rates are not completely understood, but some explanations include the following [9]:

1. Women are having fewer children; thus, a greater percentage of births are among nulliparous, who are at increased risk for caesarean delivery.

2. The average maternal age is rising, and older women, especially nulliparous, have a higher risk of caesarean delivery.

3. The use of electronic foetal monitoring is widespread. This practice is associated with an increased caesarean delivery rate compared with intermittent foetal heart rate auscultation. Foetal distress accounts for only a minority of all caesarean deliveries. In many more cases, concern for an abnormal or "non-reassuring" foetal heart rate tracing prompts caesarean delivery.
4. Most foetuses presenting breech are now delivered by caesarean section.
5. The frequency of operative vaginal delivery has declined.
6. Rates of labour induction continue to rise, and induced labour, especially among nulliparous, raises the caesarean delivery rate.
7. Obesity, which is a caesarean delivery risk, has reached epidemic proportions.
8. Rates of caesarean delivery in women with preeclampsia have increased, whereas labour induction rates for these patients have declined.
9. The rate of vaginal birth after caesarean (VBAC) has decreased.
10. Elective caesarean deliveries are increasingly being performed for various indications that include maternal request, concern for pelvic floor injury associated with vaginal birth and reduction of foetal injury rates.
11. Assisted reproductive technology is more widely used than in the past and is associated with greater caesarean delivery rates.
12. Malpractice litigation related to foetal injury during spontaneous or operative vaginal delivery continues to contribute to the present caesarean delivery rate.
13. Fear of birth and labour pain.
14. Belief that caesarean section prevents trauma and damage to the pelvic due to vaginal birth.
15. Belief that caesarean section is less traumatic to the baby.
16. Convenience to the care provider and mother.
17. Low tolerance of anything less than perfect birth outcome.
18. Cultural considerations, e.g. birth date being lucky for future or destiny.

Looking at the different caesarean section rates across the globe, it appears mothers around the world end up with less than optimal care when it comes to caesarean sections. It is either too little too late or too much too soon.

8. Robson's classification for CS

As already discussed, there are concerns over the rising caesarean section rate globally. However, determining the adequate caesarean section rate at the population level, i.e. the minimum rate for medically indicated caesarean section, while avoiding medically unnecessary operations is a challenging task. At the heart of the challenge in defining the optimal caesarean section rate at any level is the lack of a reliable and internationally accepted classification system to produce standardised data, enabling comparisons across populations and providing a tool to investigate drivers of the upward trend in caesarean section.

The lack of a standardised internationally accepted classification system to monitor and compare caesarean section rates in a consistent and action-oriented manner is one of the factors that has hindered a better understanding of this trend. WHO proposes adopting Robson's classification as an internationally applicable caesarean section classification system [29].

The system classifies all women admitted for delivery into 1 of the 10 groups that are mutually exclusive and totally inclusive. This means that based on a few basic obstetric variables, every woman admitted to deliver in any facility can be classified into 1, and only 1, of the 10 groups and no woman will be left out of the classification. The 10 groups are based on 6 basic obstetric variables which are the only information needed to classify each woman as shown in **Table 2**.

Based on the 6 obstetrics, the 10 groups are as shown in **Table 3**.

WHO expects that this classification will help healthcare facilities to:

1. Optimise the use of caesarean section by identifying, analysing and focusing interventions on specific groups of particular relevance for each healthcare facility.

2. Assess the effectiveness of strategies or interventions targeted at optimising the use of caesarean section.

3. Assess the quality of care, clinical management practices and outcomes by group.

4. Assess the quality of the data collected while raising staff awareness about the importance of the data and its use.

Obstetric characteristic	
1. Parity	• Nulliparous • Multiparous
2. Previous caesarean section	• Yes (one or more) • No
3. Onset of labour	• Spontaneous • Induced • No labour (prelabour caesarean section)
4. Number of foetuses	• Singleton • Multiple
5. Gestational age	• Preterm (less than 37 weeks) • Term (37 weeks or more)
6. Foetal lie and presentation	• Cephalic presentation • Breech presentation • Transverse lie

Reproduced from WHO Robson classification implementation manual 2017.

Table 2.
Obstetric variables for Robson's classification.

Group	Description
Group 1	Nulliparous women with a single cephalic pregnancy ≥37 weeks gestation in spontaneous labour
Group 2	Nulliparous women with a single cephalic pregnancy, ≥37 weeks gestation who either had labour induced or were delivered by caesarean section before labour
Group 3	Multiparous women without a previous uterine scar, with a single cephalic pregnancy ≥37 weeks gestation in a spontaneous labour
Group 4	Multiparous women without a previous uterine scar, with a single cephalic pregnancy ≥37 weeks gestation who either had labour induced or were delivered by caesarean section before labour
Group 5	All multiparous women with at least one previous uterine scar with a single cephalic pregnancy ≥37 weeks gestation
Group 6	All nulliparous women with a single breech pregnancy
Group 7	All multiparous women with a single breech pregnancy, including women with previous uterine scar
Group 8	All women with multiple pregnancies, including women with previous uterine scars
Group 9	All women with a single pregnancy with a transverse or oblique lie, including women with previous uterine scar
Group 10	All women with a single cephalic pregnancy <37 weeks, including women with previous uterine scar

Reproduced from WHO Robson classification implementation manual 2017.

Table 3.
The 10 groups of the Robson classification.

9. Conclusion

Caesarean sections are effective in saving maternal and infant lives but only when they are required for medically indicated reasons. Although the operation continues to become safer, the incidence of maternal mortality and morbidity is still significant. Continued efforts on the part of the obstetrician must be made to ensure that caesarean deliveries are not performed for inappropriate indications and that each woman is counselled carefully according to her individual characteristics. Caesarean section rates have been rising over time due to multifactorial reasons. However, determining the adequate caesarean section rate is challenging due to the absence of reliable and internationally accepted classification system. WHO proposes Robson's classification system as a global standard for assessing, monitoring and comparing caesarean section rates within healthcare facilities and between facilities. However, every effort should be made to provide caesarean sections to women in need, rather than striving to achieve a specific caesarean section rate.

Author details

Josaphat Byamugisha* and Moses Adroma
Department of Obstetrics and Gynaecology, School of Medicine, College of Health Sciences Makerere University, Kampala, Uganda

*Address all correspondence to: jbyamugisha@gmail.com

References

[1] Louis HS. Cesarean Delivery. Medscape; 2018. Available from: https://emedicine.medscape.com/article/263424-overview

[2] Gabert HA, Bey M. History and development of cesarean operation. Obstetrics and Gynecology Clinics of North America. 1988;**15**(4):591-605

[3] Naji O, Abdallah Y, et al. Cesarean birth: Surgical techniques. The Global Library of Women's Medicine; 2010. ISSN: 1756-2228. DOI: 10.3843/GLOWM.10133

[4] Tungshevinsirikul R et al. Advanced abdominal pregnancy: A case report. Journal of the Medical Association of Thailand. 1990;**73**(Suppl 1):107-110

[5] Shojai R et al. Advanced combined abdominal and intrauterine pregnancy: A case report. Fetal Diagnosis and Therapy. 2007;**22**(2):128-130

[6] TODMAN D. A history of caesarean section: From ancient world to the modern era. Australian and New Zealand Journal of Obstetrics and Gynaecology. 2007;**47**(5):357-361

[7] Boley JP. The history of caesarean section. 1935. CMAJ: Canadian Medical Association Journal = Journal de l'Association Medicale Canadienne. 1991;**145**(4):319-322

[8] Vincenzo Berghella M. Cesarean Delivery: Preoperative Planning and Patient Preparation. Uptodate; 2018. Available from: https://www.uptodate.com/contents/cesarean-delivery-preoperative-planning-and-patient-preparation/print

[9] Cunningham FG. Williams Obstetrics. In: Cunningham FG, Leveno KJ, Bloom SL, Dashe JS, Hoffman BL, Casey BM, Spong CY, et al, editors. 25th ed. McGraw-Hill Education; 2018

[10] Alfirevic Z, Milan SJ, Livio S. Caesarean section versus vaginal delivery for preterm birth in singletons. Cochrane Database of Systematic Reviews. 2012;(6):Cd000078

[11] How HY et al. Is vaginal delivery preferable to elective cesarean delivery in fetuses with a known ventral wall defect? American Journal of Obstetrics and Gynecology. 2000;**182**(6):1527-1534

[12] Friedman AM et al. Gastroschisis: Epidemiology and mode of delivery, 2005-2013. American Journal of Obstetrics and Gynecology. 2016;**215**(3):348.e1-348.e3489

[13] Lyerly AD et al. Risks, values, and decision making surrounding pregnancy. Obstetrics and Gynecology. 2007;**109**(4):979-984

[14] Story L, Paterson-Brown S. Cesarean deliveries: Indications, techniques and complications. In: Warren R, Arulkumaran S, editors. Chapter 10. Best Practice in Labour and Delivery. Cambridge University Press; 2009

[15] Lucas DN et al. Urgency of caesarean section: A new classification. Journal of the Royal Society of Medicine. 2000;**93**(7):346-350

[16] Ingram GS. The lessons of the national confidential enquiry into perioperative deaths. Best Practice & Research Clinical Anaesthesiology. 1999;**13**(3):257-266

[17] Berghella V, Baxter JK, Chauhan SP. Evidence-based surgery for cesarean delivery. American Journal of Obstetrics and Gynecology. 2005;**193**(5):1607-1617

[18] Holmgren G, Sjoholm L, Stark M. The Misgav Ladach method for cesarean section: Method description. Acta Obstetricia et Gynecologica Scandinavica. 1999;**78**(7):615-621

[19] Wood RM, Simon H, Oz AU. Pelosi-type vs. traditional cesarean delivery. A prospective comparison. The Journal of Reproductive Medicine. 1999;**44**(9):788-795

[20] Shipp TD et al. Intrapartum uterine rupture and dehiscence in patients with prior lower uterine segment vertical and transverse incisions. Obstetrics and Gynecology. 1999;**94**(5 Pt 1):735-740

[21] Yazicioglu F et al. Incomplete healing of the uterine incision after caesarean section: Is it preventable? European Journal of Obstetrics, Gynecology, and Reproductive Biology. 2006;**124**(1):32-36

[22] Vincenzo Berghella M. Cesarean Delivery: Technique. Uptodate; 2018. Available from: https://www.uptodate.com/contents/cesarean-delivery-surgical-technique

[23] Cheong YC et al. To close or not to close? A systematic review and a meta-analysis of peritoneal non-closure and adhesion formation after caesarean section. European Journal of Obstetrics, Gynecology, and Reproductive Biology. 2009;**147**(1):3-8

[24] Chelmow D, Rodriguez EJ, Sabatini MM. Suture closure of subcutaneous fat and wound disruption after cesarean delivery: A meta-analysis. Obstetrics and Gynecology. 2004; **103**(5 Pt 1):974-980

[25] Mackeen AD, Berghella V, Larsen ML. Techniques and materials for skin closure in caesarean section. Cochrane Database of Systematic Reviews. 2012;(9):Cd003577

[26] Clay FS, Walsh CA, Walsh SR. Staples vs subcuticular sutures for skin closure at cesarean delivery: A metaanalysis of randomized controlled trials. American Journal of Obstetrics and Gynecology. 2011;**204**(5):378-383

[27] Frishman GN, Schwartz T, Hogan JW. Closure of Pfannenstiel skin incisions. Staples vs. subcuticular suture. The Journal of Reproductive Medicine. 1997;**42**(10):627-630

[28] Berghella V. Cesarean Delivery: Postoperative Issues. Uptodate; 2018. Available from: https://www.uptodate.com/contents/cesarean-delivery-postoperative-issues

[29] WHO H. WHO WHO Statement on Caesarean Section Rates. 2015

[30] Ye J, Betrán AP, Guerrero Vela M, Souza JP, Zhang J. Searching for the optimal rate of medically necessary cesarean delivery. Birth. 2014;**41**(3):237-244

[31] Mi J, Liu F. Rate of caesarean section is alarming in China. Lancet. 2014;**383**(9927):1463-1464

[32] Nakamura-Pereira M et al. Use of Robson classification to assess cesarean section rate in Brazil: The role of source of payment for childbirth. Reproductive Health. 2016;**13**(Suppl 3):128-128